PLAY IN HOSPITALS

Exploring how practitioners make use of play's developmental benefits and therapeutic healing properties to aid the child's healthcare journey, this reflective book expands and enhances the knowledge base underlying the practice of play in hospitals.

The work of health play specialists and child life specialists in hospitals in the UK and around the world requires a deep level of clinical knowledge, so that preparing children for procedures can be done with skill and precision. It builds on an understanding of both child development and the impact of traumatic experiences so that children's deepest fears and biggest emotions can be faced without flinching. It also relies on an acceptance that play is the foundation of everything – the child's safest, most natural space – and from this trust, strength and resilience can grow and be nurtured. This new edited text explores the breadth, depth and skills of these trained healthcare practitioners providing play for babies, children, young people and adults, and places the power of play squarely at the centre of most clinical settings. Its starting point of the theory that underpins practice is explored and developed through a combination of reflective essays, case study chapters from the UK and around the world and the newly emerging use of play in diverse settings.

Drawing on the collective work of over 30 play specialists, child life specialists, play service managers, lecturers and researchers, this book is unique in all it offers to paediatric practitioners and settings, in training and in practice. It is an important resource for healthcare play specialists, playworkers, children's nurses, occupational therapists and more.

Nicky Everett is a Senior Lecturer on the Childhood Development and Playwork course at Leeds Beckett University and Health Play Specialist. Previous to her role at the University, Nicky was employed for just over 14 years at the Leeds

Teaching Hospital Trust (NHS). Working within Paediatric Oncology, her role involved normalising play where possible for her patients, along with guiding children and young people through a variety of procedures, such as CT and MRI scans, blood tests and chemotherapy. Staying within oncology, her role then moved over to be a Teenage Cancer Trust, Youth Support Coordinator within the teenage and young adult team working with young people aged between 13 and 18 years. Outside of the Oncology Team, Nicky was also involved in helping set up the Leeds Children's Hospital Youth Forum. Nicky is passionate about the role of play within a hospital setting for both children and young people and is currently focusing on this aspect within her role at the University.

Cath Hubbuck is a registered Senior Health Play Specialist. She studied BSc Early Childhood Studies at Bristol University and qualified as a HPS in 2001. Cath has worked in a number of hospitals around the UK. She is currently based at Great Ormond Street Hospital for Children in London where she is a senior member of the hospital's play team. Cath is the author of *Play for Sick Children: Play Specialists in Hospital and Beyond*. She has delivered teaching on the FdA Healthcare Play Specialism training course, and spoken at national and international conferences on subjects including the importance of normalising play as part of the HPS's role, and theoretical approaches to understanding children's lived experiences of illness and treatment. Cath has worked within various clinical specialities, including Burns and Plastics, Outpatients, Oncology and PICU. Cath is keen to develop a collective understanding within the HPS profession of hospital-associated trauma and its short and longer effects on children and families

Fraser Brown, PhD, was the first Professor of Playwork in the UK. He was Director of Studies for all postgraduate play, play therapy and playwork research at Leeds Beckett University, and specialist link tutor for the postgraduate play therapy courses run in conjunction with the Academy of Play and Child Psychotherapy. He is well known for his research into the therapeutic impact of playwork on a group of abandoned children in a Romanian paediatric hospital. He was the founder and Chair of the Aid for Romanian Children Charitable Trust (ARC), which works to alleviate the plight of Roma children in Romania. His awards include the Chancellor's Award for Innovation in Education, the Playwork Writer of the Year Award and the Brian Sutton-Smith Play Scholar Award. He is Co-Editor of the *International Journal of Play*, and his recent publications include *Aspects of Playwork* (2018); *101 Stories of Children Playing* (2014); *Rethinking Children's Play* (2013); and *Foundations of Playwork* (2008).

PLAY IN HOSPITALS

Real Life Perspectives

Edited by Nicky Everett, Cath Hubbuck and Fraser Brown

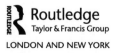
Routledge
Taylor & Francis Group

LONDON AND NEW YORK

Cover image: © Daniela Pérez-Duarte Arredondo

First published 2023
by Routledge
4 Park Square, Milton Park, Abingdon, Oxon OX14 4RN

and by Routledge
605 Third Avenue, New York, NY 10158

Routledge is an imprint of the Taylor & Francis Group, an informa business

British Library Cataloguing-in-Publication Data
A catalogue record for this book is available from the British Library

Library of Congress Cataloging-in-Publication Data
Names: Everett, Nicky, editor. | Hubbuck, Catherine, editor. |
Brown, Fraser, 1951- editor.
Title: Play in hospitals : real life perspectives / edited by
Nicky Everett, Cath Hubbuck and Fraser Brown.
Description: Milton Park, Abingdon, Oxon ; New York,
NY : Routledge, 2023. | Includes bibliographical references and index.
Identifiers: LCCN 2022049666 (print) | LCCN 2022049667
(ebook) Subjects: LCSH: Play therapy. | Children--Hospital care.
Classification: LCC RJ505.P6 P527 2023 (print) | LCC RJ505.P6
(ebook) | DDC 618.92/891653--dc23/eng/20221214
LC record available at https://lccn.loc.gov/2022049666
LC ebook record available at https://lccn.loc.gov/2022049667

ISBN: 978-1-032-18626-9 (hbk)
ISBN: 978-1-032-18625-2 (pbk)
ISBN: 978-1-003-25544-4 (ebk)

DOI: 10.4324/9781003255444

This is dedicated to the memory of the children whose lives are briefly touched on in this book – sadly, some of them are no longer with us.

The book is also dedicated to the memory of Gabi Marston, the first HPS to be employed in a UK hospital in the 1960s. Gabi died in August 2022 during the production of this book. Like others of her generation she was a pioneer – her interest in and support for the HPS profession continued right up until the end. Thank you, Gabi.

All royalties from this book go to:

Starlight Children's Foundation
www.starlight.org

CONTENTS

FIGURES

CONTRIBUTORS

Humara Bushra Ashraf is a qualified registered health play specialist in the UK. She has over 20 years' experience helping children and young people excel in varying capacities. She is currently working as a senior hospital play specialist across two London Trusts, which specialise in trauma and general paediatrics. Bushra worked in Dubai to help set up the child life department within the mental health centre of excellence. This involved detailed planning of services and deliverables such as the service running of the department and providing a positive experience for children attending a hospital appointment.

Nicky Bale is a Foundation Years consultant in Bristol with responsibility for The Bristol Standard. Her background is in teaching early years in mainstream Nursery, Reception and Key Stage 1. Nicky leads the Bristol Standard across Bristol and coordinates the involvement of the other local authorities that together form the Bristol Standard Family. She has used the Quality Improvement Framework within her own teaching and considers it to be transformational in bringing teams together as reflective communities and – in doing so – improving quality for children and families.

Lisa Beaumont is the Therapeutic and Specialised Play Manager at Leeds Children's Hospital. Lisa holds the Healthcare Play Specialist Qualification and has worked with a hospital setting for 31 years. Firstly, she started as a Play Leader, moving to a health play specialist, and then senior health play specialist, until starting her current role as Manager in 2018. Lisa is passionate about all aspects of play in hospital and the positive outcomes this has for all children's receiving treatment, her focus is to lead and continue to build an outstanding play team, ready for our new flag ship hospital in Leeds in 2026.

Jo Caseley has worked as a health play specialist at Bristol Royal Hospital for Children since 2014. Here, she has predominantly worked in the Paediatric Oncology and Haematology service and on the Children's Oncology Day Ward. Jo comes from a family of playworkers and before training to be a health play specialist had worked as a nanny, a play service manager and a Play Ranger lead across the Bristol and South Gloucestershire areas. Jo is passionate about making positive hospital experiences for children and families and improving the profession for the benefit of play teams in healthcare settings.

Katie Collis is a qualified health play specialist with 11 years' experience in the hospital play team. She graduated with Merit from Nescot in 2020 with a Foundation Degree in Healthcare Play Specialism. Katie is established in a district general and teaching hospital covering all paediatric disciplines from birth to 16 years and is passionate about improving the hospital experience for children and young people. Katie's background is in childcare and she also has experience supporting a play team in a children's hospice. Having struggled to find literature specific to Hospital Play during her degree, Katie is excited to contribute to this book sharing her experiences and best practice.

Sara Costa is a skilled Psychomotricist and a Certified Therapeutic Recreational Specialist (CTRS) with 8 years of experience in school and hospital settings. Sara is also trained in therapeutic play skills by PTUK. She is based in a children's hospital in Dubai, where she helped develop and establish the Child Life Department, under the Mental Health Centre of Excellence. She creates a safe space where children and adolescents can express themselves and work through emotional challenges using recreation and play. Armed with a deep understanding of child and adolescent development and multiple therapeutic techniques, she provides inpatient and outpatient services.

Joanne Cross is a senior health play specialist at University Hospitals Plymouth since 1999, qualifying as a health play specialist in 2001. Jo has a special interest in supporting children with additional needs and has been responsible for implementing resources to help during their hospitalisation. Jo sat on the board of the National Association of Health Play Specialists for over 10 years and was chair for 4 years. Jo also volunteered for her local children's bereavement charity Jeremiahs Journey for 14 years supporting children and families that had experienced a bereavement. Jo is passionate about improving healthcare through play.

Sarah Dransfield is an Osteosarcoma survivor. Having been diagnosed in 2012 at just 16, Sarah underwent a full year of intense Chemotherapy, a right leg above knee amputation and two major operations to remove metastatic tumours from her lungs. Since then, Sarah has learnt to walk again and gone on to do many things in her life from learning to drive and learning to sail amongst others. Sarah is also an active ambassador for two cancer charities, providing young people someone to turn to in times of need. Sarah is now a diverse model alongside working in her family's business. Sarah has been a mentor to many young people since completing her treatment in 2013 and now is a regular public speaker, talking about her experiences and spreading awareness.

Lynda Elliott is the Play Team Co-Ordinator & Outreach Play Specialist at Rainbows Hospice for Children and Young People, leading a small Play Team as well as delivering specific, therapeutic sessions in the community. She has a wealth of experience in childcare settings, from being a nanny, working in nurseries and in a short break facility for children and young people with disabilities, autism and behaviours that could be challenging to manage, before working in the hospice, and then qualifying as a play specialist in 2009. This is reflected through her involvement with the Play in Palliative Care Forum (Midlands).

Susan Fairclough has over 36 years' experience of working with children, young people, families and professionals in Healthcare, Education, Social Services and the Voluntary Sector. She has been a qualified and registered health play specialist since 1991 and Head of Play Service – therapeutic and specialised play services manager since 1998 at Royal Manchester Children's Hospital, and Youth Service Manager from 2021 for the Manchester University NHS Foundation Trust. She is responsible and accountable for all the health play specialists, play leaders and play service across three hospital sites. She is also the Events Lead, organising events and entertainment to help create positive experiences and healing environments. She has been a Trustee for Action for Sick Children and an Inspector and Advisor for the Care Quality Commission (CQC) NHS England.

Julie Fisher started working on the children's Burns and Plastics/Neurology and Neurosciences ward at Frenchay Hospital in Bristol as a Hospital Play Assistant in 2001. She qualified as a health play specialist in 2003. Before starting this work, Julie had worked in a school and undertaken the NNEB Diploma training. When Frenchay Hospital closed in 2014 the play team moved to join play colleagues at Bristol Royal Hospital for Children. Julie took up a position here as a Senior HPS. In 2018, Julie was appointed Play Manager with oversight for the whole team – a role she was overjoyed to take on and which she thoroughly enjoyed for the next four years. Julie retired in May 2022 after a 21-year career in hospital play.

Leanne Hallowell, MEd (Melb), is a Lecturer in the Faculty of Education and Arts, at Australian Catholic University, and is a PhD candidate at the University of Melbourne. She was previously Head of Educational Play Therapy at the Royal Children's Hospital, Melbourne. Leanne's work at RCH was varied, working in the emergency department, with children with cystic fibrosis, children requiring liver transplantation, and in radiology. Work in radiology included developing a programme to support children undergoing MRI scans without the use of anaesthetic. The team working on this project won state government awards for excellence in paediatric healthcare and internationally for clinical practice in radiology. Leanne's current research describes and theorises effective engagement with children in medical settings, in particular medical interventions and procedures. Leanne has also worked as a consultant with architectural firms on supportive environments in paediatric healthcare and educational settings.

Charlotte Hamflett developed a passion for play as a young person. She was fascinated to observe children making toys out of rubbish in Lesotho, and to experience the way that gestures, fun and games crossed the language barrier. Prior to qualifying as a hospital play specialist in 2003, she was privileged to spend a month with volunteers in an Eastern European orphanage, facilitating sensory stimulation to children suffering from deprivation. During a 15-year career, Charlotte has worked as a play specialist in a Paediatric A&E and in both outpatient and inpatient environments. Her professional interests include sibling support, paediatric continence, oncology and play support for children with autism, learning difficulties and sensory impairments.

Penelope Hart-Spencer, MSc, is an experienced health play specialist, specialising in oncology for over 14 years. She has worked in ICU/HDU, burns and was previously an associate lecturer at Manchester Metropolitan University. She supports children, young people and their families through their radiotherapy and proton beam therapy at The Christie Manchester (the largest single-site cancer centre in Europe). Penelope was part of the team who developed the UK's first proton beam therapy centre at The Christie in 2018. In 2016, she spent time at University of Florida Proton Therapy Institute, learning about supporting patients through proton beam therapy and this greatly informed her practice. Penelope is the chair of The National Association of Health Play Specialists. She is also registered with the Health Play Specialist Education Trust. She is a reviewer for Children's Cancer & Leukaemia Group publications and has published a children's book about hair loss and articles in academic journals relating to her work as a health play specialist.

Cala Hefferan is a certified child life specialist (CCLS) at MHealth Fairview Masonic Children's Hospital and Clinics. Cala began her career in child life as a Child Life Associate (CLA) at Children's Hospital and Clinics of Minnesota, where she gained invaluable experience designing and facilitating play experiences in the inpatient setting and a therapeutic play space specially designed for patients and their families. As a CCLS, she strives to apply evidence-based best practices as she collaborates across disciplines to integrate developmental perspectives to support paediatric patients and their families. Cala is passionate about incorporating play into child life interventions and advocating for play experiences that promote resilience.

Gemma Hookins, MA, is a Play Therapist, she is currently working at a Children's Hospital in Dubai, where she has helped to set up and run the child life department, under the mental health centre of excellence. She provides play therapy within the hospital and in the outpatient clinic. Gemma has over 20 years' experience working with children and young people, in a variety of settings in the UK and United Arab Emirates. Her background is in education, where she has worked as a special needs teacher, a class teacher, with a mixed class of Special needs and mainstream children, and a foundation stage two class teacher.

Katie Lane is a qualified and registered health play specialist, with a foundation degree in Healthcare Play Specialism and a BA (Hons) in Early Years Development with Education. Currently working at Bristol Royal Hospital for Children, the paediatric medical centre of excellence for the southwest of England. In her four years at the BRHC, she has sought to build the profile of the importance of the 'power of play' in supporting children through medical procedural interventions. Katie is passionate about advocating for children, young people and their families in the hospital setting. Her collaborations, within the play team at Bristol, have led to the team being awarded the 'Bristol Standard Quality Improvement for Play Provision Certificate' after completing the 'Bristol Standards'.

Lobke Marsden is a health play specialist based in Leeds. She has been supporting children and young people through their radiotherapy treatment over the past 18 years. She is passionate about making her patients radiotherapy treatment journey as positive as possible and is always looking for different ways to support this. One way of improving patient experience is by painting the radiotherapy masks which some patients require for their treatment, in their chosen design to make them look and feel less clinical. Lobke qualified as an art therapist in the Netherlands. The Wellcome Galleries at the Science Museum in London has one of these radiotherapy masks painted by Lobke on display for the next 25 years.

Tracey Martin is an experienced health play specialist whose hospital play career began in 1986. She worked on the Cystic Fibrosis and Respiratory ward at Leeds Teaching Hospitals between 2002 and 2021. Besides her role on a busy ward, she also worked alongside the Psychology Department, helping children with procedural anxieties. It was during this work that Tracey developed the Little PALs care pathway now used at Leeds Children's Hospital. In 2021/2022 she became one of the first play specialists to lead in active research, during a six-month study using virtual reality distraction therapy during painful procedures.

Chika Matsudaira is a mother, a wife and a researcher starting her career as a Social Worker. While working at the University of Shizuoka Junior College, she became a health play specialist and studied Adlerian Play Therapy to support children with therapeutic play. Now she manages the University's Hospital Play Specialist education course which was started in 2006 by the commission of the Ministry of Education, Culture, Sports, Science and Technology (MEXT) of Japan. Since then, more than 200 professionals have received the training to practice child-friendly medical care. Currently, she also works as an advisor for the Shizuoka City Child Protection Center and provides consulting services for residential children's homes. Her most recent book is *Asobi ni Ikiru Kodomotachi* (*Children Living in Play*).

Irene O'Donnell, BA (Hons) Reg HPSET, is the NHS Hospital Trust Lead for therapeutic play, recreation and youth services and professional lead for health play specialists at University College London Hospitals NHS Trust. A registered health play specialist for over 20 years, she has been a leader in using play as a tool to avoid the use of general anaesthesia for children and young people during procedures. She piloted the novel *MRI Awake* project, a finalist in the British Medical Journal Awards 2017, and recognised nationally in the NHS *Getting It Right First Time* radiology programme (2020). Irene was a lecturer on the hospital play specialist training course at Stanmore College (UWL) and is still involved in education on play in healthcare with a variety of organisations. She has held positions as chair and vice chair of the National Association of Health Play Specialists (NAHPS) and remains on their board of trustees, alongside a role on the board of the Healthcare Play Specialist Education Trust (HPSET).

Michael M. Patte (PhD, The Pennsylvania State University) is Professor of Teaching and Learning and Program Coordinator of the Child Life Specialist and Playwork Certificate Minor Programs, Bloomsburg University, USA. He is a Distinguished Fulbright Scholar, Co-Editor of the *International Journal of Play*, and Past President of The Association for the Study of Play. He has published several books and journal articles including *Rethinking Children's Play, Celebrating 40 years of Play Research and the Handbook of International Perspectives on Early Childhood Education*. His research interests include play, child development and fostering home, school, and community partnerships.

Barrington Powell has currently worked within the NHS Environment for over 25 years. He was one of the first professional Clown Doctors in the North-West of England, as a specialised entertainer, becoming one of the first performers within the hospital environment to work on a weekly basis. He has subsequently and successfully run his own programmes within the Trust including Manchester Children's Hospital, through *Orly's Magic*, and currently for Liverpool Alder Hey Children's Hospital. Barrington was part of an award-winning team who was asked to provide structured entertainment on the adult wards, as part of an initiative to provide help and raise awareness in light of the 'Mid Staffordshire' and 'Francis' reports, providing an insight on adult wards for Manchester, using techniques used in therapeutic and specialised play.

Ana Smith is a Senior Play Specialist at Kidz First Children's Hospital in Auckland, New Zealand where, for 18 years, she has worked predominantly in Emergency Departments. Her major contributions include research into supporting children and parents through burns dressing changes, creating a model of care for the Play Service, writing hospital guidelines including *Roles and responsibilities during a paediatric death in the Emergency Department*, and supporting children through the death of a parent in the ICU setting. She has also refined an 'on the job' Preceptorship Package for new employees to learn play specialist skills and knowledge. Ana has supported the growth of the profession by contributing to the organisation of bi-annual conferences of the Hospital Play Specialist Association of NZ/Aotearoa. She was a play specialist on an Operation Smile mission to China, worked with a medical response team post-Tsunami in Sri Lanka, worked as an outpatient play specialist in an acute London hospital, and supported over 300 children having blood tests as part of a vaccine clinical trial.

David Stonehouse, PhD, is currently Senior Lecturer in Associate Nursing at Leeds Beckett University. He joined the charity Pop-Up Adventure Play as a tutor in 2013, supporting students from around the world undertaking the Playwork Development Programme. 2020 saw David become an Associate Lecturer with the Open University supporting nursing students undertaking modules online. He regularly publishes articles in a range of subjects from professional issues, management and leadership, and play aimed at students and professionals within the clinical field.

Laura Sufka, MA, is a Certified child life specialist working in Private Practice. She is the Owner and Founder of Children's Coping Connection, LLC. Laura is passionate about play in the lives of children and youth and has worked with children and families impacted by illness and life events in her community for more than 20 years. Her work focuses on supporting patients and families with chronic illness, grief support, sibling support groups, educating staff on the importance of therapeutic play within paediatric healthcare, and emergency care and long-term coping of paediatric patients.

Mikaela Sullivan is a dually certified Therapeutic Recreation Specialist (CTRS) and Child Life Specialist (CCLS) at MHealth Fairview Masonic Children's Hospital. Mikaela has a unique interest in adaptive play, acute care and sibling support. She also facilitated a pilot of child life services in paediatric sleep medicine, resulting in published evidence in support of child life services: *A Certified Child Life Specialist Influences the Emotional Response During Polysomnography Setup (2022)*. Mikaela is currently in a role establishing child life services for the first time in the neonatal intensive care unit, supporting patients, siblings and families navigating long-term hospitalisation and chronic illness. She is an integrated member of the medical team and a consistent advocate for establishing normalcy in the hospital environment, building resiliency and coping skills for patients and families during medical events.

Nicola Voos is a qualified and registered health play specialist, HPSET Board member and FE Teacher in Health, Social and Childcare. Nicola did the BTEC National Diploma in Childhood Studies and worked in a day nursery where she undertook the Special Educational Needs Co-ordinator (SENCo) role and completed the NCFE Special Needs Assistance Certificate. She went on to become a play leader at Royal Manchester Children's Hospital, qualifying as a health play specialist in 2003. In 2019 Nicola gained her level 5 Education and Training Award in Further Education. Nicola plans to continue working in FE and aspires to work in a SEND college in the future.

Judy Walker is a subject matter expert in the After Action Review approach to team learning now working for a private company (iTS Leadership Ltd) after 34 years employed in the National Health Service. From 1984 to 2008 Judy worked as first a Hospital Play Specialist (HPS) and then as a Hospital Play Services Manager, growing the play service within the University College London Hospital from one person to 18 HPS. Clinically, she pioneered the role of the HPS in the Radiotherapy Department, dental hospital setting and Neonatal Unit and established a professional management structure integrated within the Paediatric Department. Judy was an active member of National Executive Committee of the National Association of Hospital Play Staff for 21 years, acting the editor of the HPS Journal and was Chair for 7 years.

Laura Walsh is the Head of Play at the Starlight Foundation. She was formerly Head of Play at Great Ormond Street Hospital for Children in Central London, leading a team of health play specialists and playworkers to support children and young people from the UK and internationally, with a wide variety of conditions which require specialist treatment. Through advocating for play as the dominant narrative in paediatric services the team focus on making explicit children's right and freedom to play and engage with their diagnosis and treatment in a way which suits them. Laura previously led the children and young people services at Central YMCA ensuring children and young people in central London could explore their own interests in their own way.

Tracy West is currently an Oncology Outreach Play Specialist working within the Children's Cancer Outreach team at Leeds General Infirmary. She has devoted her professional career to improving the hospital experience of children she has worked with. More recently she has had the privilege opportunity to establish a play specialist role based within the Macmillan team. The role is funded by Candlelighters children's charity and gives her the flexibility to work with children within their own home where they feel safe and in control. She is passionate about looking beyond the hospital and the effects of having a serious illness and bereavement on the families particularly siblings.

Mike Wragg, PhD, is Senior Lecturer in Childhood Development and Playwork at Leeds Beckett University, and Chair of Trustees of two children's play projects: Play Bradford and New Hall Prison Visitors' Play Facility. He has experience as both a practitioner and a manager of play projects. His doctoral research looks at the role of play in the creative industries, and he has spoken on this subject at national and international conferences.

ACKNOWLEDGEMENTS

Nicky would like to say a huge thank you to all the contributors within this book; without them this would not have been possible. I am sure each one of them will be happy to be free of my regular emails! To my family and friends for their constant support and encouragement, especially Aimee and Lucie. And finally thank you to Cath and Fraser for taking on this journey with me ... We did it!

Cath would like to thank so many health play colleagues – those who have brilliantly recreated an insight into their professional work in these chapters and all those who have made my own workdays such a joy over many years. Thank you Laura, Sian and Demi for being there on my 'Angry HPS' days! Special thanks to Jessica for reminding me of just how valuable play – and friendship – is for sick children. As ever, thank you to the lovely Dom for his enduring patience and support – and also to Tara, Jonathan, Peter and Hattie. x

Fraser would like to thank the contributors to the book – their patience with my pedantic editing has been amazing. I should also like to thank colleagues and students at Leeds Beckett University for their dedication and commitment to the Playwork course and for the inspiration they provide on a daily basis. Finally, I want to thank my family and friends for their patience and support. They may have expected something different when I decided to retire. So, thank you as always to Anne, Louisa, James, Lucy and Emily.

The editors would like to thank Daniela Pérez-Duarte Arredondo for creating the cover art for this book.

GLOSSARY

NB. Health play specialist, hospital play specialist, healthcare play specialist and child life specialist are descriptors that are used interchangeably throughout this book, depending on the preference and/or location of particular contributors.

CAT Scan	computerised axial tomography scan (sometimes just CT Scan)
CLS	child life specialist
CYP	children and young people
GA	general anaesthetic
HPS	may refer to health play specialist, hospital play specialist or healthcare play specialist
HPSET	Healthcare Play Specialist Education Trust
ICU	Intensive Care Unit
IPA	International Play Association
MDT	multidisciplinary team
MRI	magnetic resonance imaging
NAHPS	National Association of Health Specialists
NHS	National Health Service
NICE	National Institute for Health and Care Excellence
NSF	National Service Framework for Children
SCF	Save the Children Fund
UNCRC	United Nations Convention on the Rights of the Child
WRI	White Rose Initiative

INTRODUCTION

Fraser Brown – Emeritus Professor of Playwork

Mike Wragg – Senior Lecturer in Childhood Development and Playwork

The subject of play has long been regarded by those who take an academic interest in it as one that is so notoriously ambiguous and open to interpretation that it evades definition (Sutton-Smith, 1997). As Brockman et al. (2011) point out, there is a distinct lack of agreement amongst academics when attempting to reach an overarching definition; so much so that Smith et al. (2019) suggest many researchers have virtually given up attempting to define the subject. It is, in part, argued that this is because the documented benefits of play are so multitudinous, and relatable to virtually all aspects of human growth and development, that they are too vast to be captured by a single description (Sandseter, 2011).

However, according to Zosh et al. (2017), the process by which the benefits of play are derived is marked by a number of common characteristics. These include experimentation, exploration, boundary testing, personal choice and control, intrinsic motivation, freedom to fail, positive affect, flexibility, and adaptation. For example, according to Resnick (2017), through processes of hypothesis testing, play is associated with enhanced divergent thought processes, which Winnicott (1971) says enhances creativity.

Play and creativity are closely related in the literature, for example Bateson (2014) suggests elements of play such as risk-taking, problem-solving, imagination, and exploration replicate essential processes of creativity. Play involving creativity and problem solving is associated with what Scult et al. (2019) refer to as higher-order executive brain functions. Such functions include empathetic thinking (Craft, 2013); the ability to imagine one's future self (Gotlieb et al., 2019); emotional resilience and self-regulation (Vitalaki et al., 2017); and inter-subjectivity (Sawyer, 2012). A study by Harvard University's Centre on the Developing Child associates these higher-order functions with the deferred benefits of increased future earning potential and improved physical and mental health in adulthood (NSCDC, 2007).

DOI: 10.4324/9781003255444-1

The immediate benefits of play to children's physical and mental health and well-being are also particularly well documented in the literature. For example, a comprehensive study by Ignjatovic et al. (2019) identified play as a contributing factor in increased bone mineral density, cardio-respiratory fitness, and enhanced mental health. In further relation to mental health, play is identified as a protective factor for well-being (Gilham, 2018), and the notion of play as an inherently healing behaviour is also well established (Jennings & Holmwood, 2021). Matthews and Rix (2013), relate this to the players' enhanced sense of autonomy, which Purswell and Taylor (2013) associate with the development of complex emotional coping strategies. According to Edwards (2016), play stimulates the production of what are often popularly referred to as 'happy' or 'feel-good' hormones, such as endorphins, oxytocin, dopamine, and serotonin, which are associated with feelings of pleasure, reward, and motivation.

Given this holistic array of physical and psychological benefits, it is unsurprising that a deficit of play is correlated negatively with children's healthy development and well-being. According to Hughes (2003) too little developmentally critical play can result in biological and social disablement. This condition, referred to in the literature as play deprivation (Pellis & Pellis, 2017), is associated with adverse physical and mental health outcomes (Alexander et al., 2014) and has also been identified as a source of chronic physical and cognitive retardation and psychosis (Brown, 2009).

As we emerge from an unprecedented period of social restrictions as a consequence of the COVID-19 pandemic, an increasing number of studies drawing attention to the detrimental consequences of restrictions on play and social interaction for children's health and well-being have come to the fore (e.g. UNICEF, 2022). This has led to a growing prominence of calls for more play for children to attenuate these harmful outcomes (Weale, 2021). Over the course of the last generation, a decline in play opportunities has affected all children across much of the Western world (Whitebread, 2017). This decline is associated with a number of factors including risk-averse parenting approaches (Wodda, 2018), the commercialisation of play, and the pressures of academic achievement at increasingly younger ages (Brooker & Woodhead, 2013).

For children who are unwell or have chronic illnesses, restricted access to the holistic benefits of play is particularly pronounced, and yet we know that play for these children can offer additional benefits to health, development, and well-being (Tonkin, 2014). For example, children's self-reported experiences of play illustrate that it helps them overcome the isolating effects of hospitalisation (Weil, 2013). Furthermore, stress and anxiety associated with needle phobia can be reduced by exploring these feelings through play (Jelbert et al., 2005). Play in hospital is also known to alleviate boredom (Aldiss et al., 2009) and enable children to build resilience and develop coping strategies across the age range (Gleave & Cole-Hamilton, 2012).

This book, the first of its kind to bring together the experiences of practitioners using the medium of play with ill and hospitalised children, explores the methods, techniques, and benefits of this under-researched and vital intervention in children's lives. Of course, great strides have been made in this field in the last 50 years. In the UK it is not so long ago that the following situation was an accepted norm.

FRASER'S RECOLLECTION

I had four operations before the age of four to correct the facial disfigurement I had been born with. On each occasion I was taken to the hospital and collected two weeks later by my parents. They had no telephone, and I had no contact with them during that whole time. So, why am I not a deeply traumatised person?

I am in no doubt about the answer to that question. In those days the nurses saw their role holistically. In other words, the nurses played with me.

Gradually, in the intervening years nurse training has become more and more medicalised. Today's children's nurses are far better qualified to deal with the medical side of a paediatric ward. However, as David Stonehouse's research shows, today's children's nurses are far too 'busy' to play with their patients. The need for Health Play Specialists to fill the void is well argued by the contributors to Part I of the book. Judy Walker explains the way in which the HPS's role has developed in recent years; and Charlotte Hamflett provides an example of a positive approach supporting the siblings of children undergoing long-term treatment programmes. Irene O'Donnell argues HPSs should be seen as a cost-effective element within the hospital environment. On the other hand, Cath Hubbuck and Joanne Cross suggest the misguided priorities of many hospitals mean they still offer essentially deprived environments for children. In particular, Irene O'Donnell describes child mental health provision as the 'elephant in the room'.

In Part II we offer a number of very personal reflections on the HPS role, starting with Lisa Beaumont's individual journey, Katie Lane's focus on 'play and distraction, and Katie Collis's 'day in the life'. In Chapter 11, Susan Fairclough explores the specialised nature of a lot of the HPS's work, while Nicky Everett highlights the 'forgotten' age group, i.e. teenagers, who have their own distinctive culture – too old to be comfortable on children's wards, but too young to be placed safely on adult wards. Finally, Cath Hubbuck explores her 'anger' and 'sadness' at the casual disrespect with which children are often treated in our hospitals. The following story illustrates the dangers of ignoring the fact that children are human beings with fundamental rights, deserving of respect.

PAULINA PÉREZ-DUARTE MENDIOLA
Clinical Paediatrician and Medical Anthropologist

I ran to the operating-room; the patient was already under anaesthesia, I asked, again, this time directly to the surgeon:

"Doctor, did you tell the child you were going to amputate two of his limbs?"

Harshly, he replied: *"That is not my job, nor my responsibility!"*

This is exactly where I was when my career, as a clinical paediatrician, turned on its head. A 12-year-old child had been admitted to the Paediatric Intensive Care Burns Unit with a serious electrical burn, which compromised the integrity of two of his limbs. Both required amputation in order to preserve his life.

My 24-hour shift had begun just as the plastic surgeon was transferring the patient to the operating room. I asked the nurses and his family-members:

"Did someone explain to the patient that he is going to have a double-amputation?" A long and disturbing silence was the answer to my query. This is when I ran to the operating room and my career changed, forever.

Ever since that experience, I have been wondering who has the 'job' or the 'responsibility' to explain procedures and chronic-illnesses to children. That day, with that specific patient, I decided to undertake the 'responsibility' as my own. Unfortunately, I was dumbfounded; I realised I had no idea how to explain procedures and chronic-illnesses to children, and nor did any of the other paediatric hospital-staff around me. So ... I tried to deliver this unique explanation as best as I knew how. This was the beginning of my professional journey, searching for answers to what I believe is a significant gap in our overall medical knowledge.

After a decade working as a clinical paediatrician, with my mind overflowing with questions and a longing to generate positive change within paediatric-healthcare, I moved to London, to study a Master's in Medical Anthropology. This is where, almost by chance, I bumped into these unsung heroes: Health Play Specialists. That is where I discovered 'specialised play' and 'imagination'. This was a watershed moment in my life and professional career. At last, I had found the professionals who have the *job* and *responsibility* to explain procedures and chronic-illnesses to children. These heroes and their work are the reason I am a 'Play and Health' researcher and advocate.

The case studies in Part III cover a range of specific areas where HPSs work, including radiotherapy treatment (Lobke Marsden), autism (Nicola Voos and Susan Fairclough), using virtual reality as a distraction technique (Tracey Martin), and the unique challenges of integrating autistic youngsters into the hospital environment. Penelope Hart–Spencer explores the role of HPSs in the care of children and young people with cancer, while the experience of teenagers in an oncology ward is given a personal twist in a 'conversation' between Nicky Everett (the HPS) and Sarah Dransfield (the patient). Rounding off this section of the book we have a couple of managerial perspectives. Firstly, Julie Fisher (play manager), Nicky Bale (consultant), and Jo Casely (HPS) summarise their experience of implementing the Bristol Standard, with the aim of embedding a more reflective approach within the hospital play team, and at the same time providing supportive evidence for their work. Finally, Laura Walsh provides a very honest reflection of what it was like to manage a play team through the Covid crisis.

The main geographical focus of this book is the UK. However, Part IV provides a selection of international perspectives. Ana Smith offers a personal view of a play specialist's journey in New Zealand, and Leanne Hallowell sets out the historical development of play in an Australian hospital. Michael Patte summarises the way in which the child life specialist approach has been incorporated into North American hospitals; while Chika Matsudaira explores the problems faced when trying to integrate HPS play in Japan. Cala Hefferan and Laura Sufka make the case for play being the best intervention tool in American Emergency Departments. Finally, Bushra Ashraf (HPS) and Gemma Hookins (play therapist) reflect on the way in which they integrated their professional skills within a hospital in the UAE.

Part V expands the boundaries to look at the way in which play is used in other ways and other settings. Lynda Elliot provides an insight into her use of play in a hospice setting. Fraser Brown reflects on the work of a therapeutic playwork project in a Romanian paediatric hospital. Irene O'Donnell explores the potential for the HPS approach to benefit adults in healthcare settings. Barrington Powell offers a number of moving accounts of his work as a 'clown doctor' in oncology wards. Cala Hefferan and Mikaela Sullivan consider the therapeutic power of play for the siblings of paediatric patients; and Tracy West shows the possibilities of taking hospital play into the home.

Taking all this together, we hope to provide insights into the work of those who use play to work with children in healthcare settings. We also hope to challenge a number of preconceptions about the importance of play, especially in hospital settings, where it is often given a very low priority. Today's hospital authorities often recognise its 'medical' value in distraction work and preparing children for procedures, but rarely do we see much recognition of the fact that children need to play to get better. Consequently, play is not a significant element in the training of children's nurses, and hospital playrooms are often misused by those who should know better. The child's right to play is enshrined in Article 31 the UNCRC. It is time our hospital authorities gave that right the recognition it deserves.

References

Aldiss, S., Hortsman, M., O'Leary, C., Richardson, A. and Gibson, F. (2009) What is important to young children who have cancer while in hospital? *Children and Society*, 23, pp. 85–98.

Alexander, S., Frohlich, K., and Fusco, C. (2019) *Play, Physical Activity and Public Health. The Reframing of Children's Leisure Lives.* London: Routledge.

Bateson, P. (2014) Play, playfulness, creativity and innovation. *Animal Behavior and Cognition,* 1(2), pp. 99–112.

Brockman, R., Jago, R. and Fox, K. (2011) What is the meaning and nature of active play for today's children in the UK? *International Journal of Behavioural Nutrition and Physical Activity,* 8(15), pp. 1–7.

Brooker, E. and Woodhead, M. (2013). *Early Childhood in Focus 9: The Right to Play.* [Online]. Available from: <http://oro.open.ac.uk/38679/1/ECIF9The Right to Play.pdf> [Accessed 14 February 2020].

Brown, S. (2009) *Play. How It Shapes the Brain, Opens the Imagination and Invigorates the Soul.* London: Penguin Books Ltd.

Craft, A. (2013). Childhood, possibility thinking and education futures. *International Journal of Education Research,* 61, pp. 126–134.

Edwards, D. (2016) *Play and the Feel Good Hormones.* [Online]. Available from: <https://www.primalplay.com/blog/play-and-the-feel-good-hormones> [Accessed 8 January 2020].

Gilham, T. (2018). Enhancing public mental health and wellbeing through creative arts participation. *Journal of Public Mental Health,* 17(4), pp. 148–156.

Gleave, J. and Cole-Hamilton, I. (2012) *A World without Play: A Literature Review.* Play England.

Gotlieb, R. Hyde, E., Immordino-Yang, M. and Kaufman, S. (2019) Imagination Is the Seed of Creativity. In: Kaufman, J. and Sternberg, R. eds. *The Cambridge Handbook of Creativity.* 2nd ed. New York City, NY: Cambridge University Press, pp. 709–731.

Hughes, B. (2003) Play deprivation and bias. In: Brown, F. ed. *Playwork Theory and Practice.* Buckingham: Open University Press, pp. 66–80.

Ignjatovic, A., Ferreira, T. and Pereira, B. (2019) Resistance Exercises or Free Play in Function of Preschool Children Inactivity Prevention. In: Antala, B., Demirhan, G., Carraro, A., Oktar, C., Oz, H. and Kaplánová, A. eds. *Physical Education in Early Childhood Education and Care Researches – Best Practices – Situation.* Bratislava: Slovak Scientific Society for Physical Education and Sport and FIEP, pp. 271–281.

Jelbert, R., Caddy, G., Mortimer, J. and Frampton, I. (2005) Procedure preparation works! An open trial of twenty four children with needle phobia or anticipatory anxiety. *The Journal of the National Association of Hospital Play Staff,* (36), pp. 14–18.

Jennings, S. and Holmwood, C. (2021) *Routledge International Handbook of Play, Therapeutic Play and Play Therapy.* London: Routledge.

Matthews, A. and Rix, J. (2013) Early intervention: Parental involvement, child agency and participation in creative play. *Early Years: An International Research Journal,* 33(3), pp. 239–251.

NSCDC (2007) *The Science of Early Childhood Development: Closing the Gap Between What We Know and What We Do.* National Scientific Council on the Developing Child [Online] Available from: <https://www.developingchild.harvard.edu> [Accessed 11 April 2021].

Pellis, S. and Pellis, V. (2017) What is play fighting and what is it good for? *Learning and Behavior,* 45(4), pp. 355–366.

Purswell, K. and Taylor, D. (2013). Creative use of sibling play therapy: An example of a blended family. *Journal of Creativity in Mental Health,* 8, pp. 162–174.

Resnick, M. (2017) *Cultivating Creativity through Projects, Passion, Peers and Play.* Cambridge, MA: MIT Press.

Sandseter, E. B. H. (2011) Children's risky play from an evolutionary perspective: The anti-phobic effects of thrilling experiences. *Evolutionary Psychology,* 9(2), pp. 257–284.

Sawyer, K. (2012). *Explaining Creativity: The Science of Human Innovation.* New York, NY: Oxford University Press.

Scult, M. A., Knodt, A. R., Radtke, S. R., Brigidi, B. D. and Hariri, A. R. (2019) Prefrontal executive control rescues risk for anxiety associated with high threat and low reward brain function. *Cerebral Cortex*, 29(1), pp. 70–76.

Smith, P. K., Takhvar, M., Gore, N. and Vollstedt, R. (2019) Play in Young Children: Problems of definition, categorization and measurement. In: Smith, P. K. ed. *Children's Play Research Developments and Practical Applications.* London: Routledge.

Sutton-Smith, B. (1997) *The Ambiguity of Play.* Cambridge, MA: Harvard University Press.

Tonkin, A. (2014) *The Provision of Play in Health Service Delivery, Fulfilling Children's Rights Under Article 31 of the United Nations Convention on the Rights of the Child.* [Online]. Available from: < https://www.england.nhs.uk/6cs/wp-content/uploads/sites/25/2015/03/nahps-full-report.pdf> [Accessed 18 July 2022].

UNICEF (2022) *Life in Lockdown Child and Adolescent Mental Health and Well-being in the Time of COVID-19.* [Online]. Available from: <http://unicef-irc.org/publications/pdf/Life-in-Lockdown.pdf> [Accessed 25 February 2022].

Vitalaki, E., Kourkoutas, E. and Hart, A. (2017). Building inclusion and resilience in students with and without SEN through the implementation of narrative speech, role play and creative writing in the mainstream classroom of primary education. *International Journal of Inclusive Education*, 22(12), 1306–1319.

Weale, S. (2021) Call for 'summer of play' to help English pupils recover from Covid-19 stress. *The Guardian*. [Online]. Available from: <https://www.theguardian.com/society/2021/feb/13/call-for-summer-of-play-to-help-english-pupils-recover-from-covid-stress> [Accessed 25 February 2022].

Weil, L. (2013) The voices of children and young people. In: *Annual Report of the Chief Medical Officer 2012, Our Children Deserve Better: Prevention Pays.* Department of Health, Chapter 4: pp. 1–20.

Whitebread, D. (2017) Free play and children's mental health. *The Lancet Child and Adolescent Mental Health*, 1(3), pp. 167–169.

Winnicott, D. (1971) *Playing and Reality.* London: Routledge

Wodda, A. (2018) Stranger danger! *Journal of Family Strengths*, 18(1), pp. 1–33.

Zosh, J., Hopkins, E., Jensen, H., Liu, C., Hirsh-Pasek, K., Solis, S. and Whitebread, D. (2017) *Learning through Play: A Review of the Evidence: White Paper.* The LEGO Foundation. [Online]. Available from: <https://www.legofoundation.com/media/1063/learning-through-play_web.pdf> [Accessed 13 July 2018].

PART I
Theoretical underpinning

1

THE DEVELOPMENT OF THE ROLE OF HOSPITAL PLAYWORKER

Judy Walker – Former Hospital Play Services Manager

When I first walked onto a children's ward in 1983, it was just over 20 years since the first person leading play in a London Hospital had been employed and it very much felt like I was a pioneer in an emerging profession. Whilst the matron who had employed me understood that play was an important activity for the child in hospital, she had little sense of the role of the Hospital Play Specialist (HPS) nor the potential of play to mitigate harm, and most clinical staff and parents saw play simply as a way of keeping children occupied and quiet.

Society has expectations of how a doctor or nurse will behave and we are all educated into these concepts from an early age through the books we read and TV programmes we watch. Since so few people understood what I and the other HPS employed at this time were there to do, no such expectation existed: it always had to be created. Every first interaction I had within the hospital setting meant some explanation of my role and purpose and some work to establish trust in this activity. So, if I was to enable a four-year-old child to be prepared for the blood test he needed, in a developmentally appropriate way, to reduce the potential trauma of being held down, I had to first educate staff about the value of preparation play, and negotiate for some preparation time in advance of the procedure, as well as win the trust of all involved.

With the word 'play' in my job title, while those around me were providing life-saving care and treatment, I was at the bottom of the ward hierarchy, and was told that I could not attend nursing handover because it was for uniformed staff only. This meant that I had limited access to information about patients. I vividly recall being asked to visit Laura, a nine-year-old with Leukaemia, who was being nursed on her own, in a side room. This was all I was told. In fact, she had relapsed three times and was seriously ill. I went in to visit her every day with a selection of age appropriate activities and on my third visit, whilst finishing painting a clay pot, she suddenly asked me "Am I going to die?" I can't

DOI: 10.4324/9781003255444-3

recall all of my response, but I do know that I didn't avoid the question and that we had a conversation about her fears and worries and I encouraged her to share these with her mother as well. Attendance at ward rounds and nursing handovers did become the norm eventually, and reading and reporting in the patients' notes became standard practice, but in those first years I often had to work in isolation with limited information.

Like all those who were originally employed to work as HPS, I had no role models to guide me as I was the only person doing this job in the hospital, so I had no immediate peers with whom to share ideas and experiences, which added to this sense of isolation. Yet the result was a freedom to innovate and be creative, and a strong determination to raise the profile of the child's developmental needs in the hospital (see Figure 1.1). I created opportunities to ensure the story of the value of play was regularly told in the hospital magazine, and I went to the school of nursing to teach student nurses about play in hospital. It was important

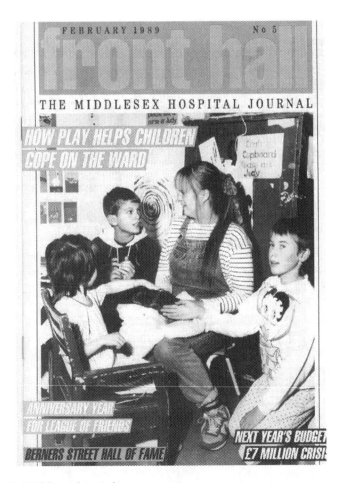

FIGURE 1.1 Middlesex hospital.

to brush off the implied criticism in the question from parents and staff, "Do you get paid to do this?" and counter it with active teaching and publicity.

The biggest challenge was to earn the right to engage with the child and family before treatment had begun so that age appropriate learning about what was to be encountered could take place, and effective coping could be enabled. Until others in the hospital understood the value of this, the standard treatment routines created for adult patients would continue and child patients would experience needless emotional harm and physical risk as a result. In my fourth year as an HPS, the Sister on my ward received a call from the Radiotherapy Superintendent, about a child who was refusing treatment and she asked if I could go and help. When I arrived in the radiotherapy department this first time, five-year-old Nicola was crying uncontrollably. Her parents were offering lots of 'bribes' to try and persuade her to lie on the treatment table and have the radiotherapy mask put on her head. This child was expected to lie still for her cranial radiation in the same way as the adults do and no one was thinking about how scary the huge machines looked to her. Nor was anyone recognising how terrifying it might feel to be left alone in a room with no idea about what would happen next. Over the next hour, I helped everyone calm down, built rapport with Nicola and her parents, as well as the radiotherapists and demonstrated what would happen using a teddy bear. As we played with the teddy in the treatment room and moved up and down the long corridor between the treatment bed and the room where the parents would be watching the treatment, Nicola gained a sense of the space and time and started to master her fears. We finally saw Nicola lie down for her own 3-minute treatment which was then able to be repeated daily for the required 30 days.

This demonstration of the benefit of using play within the Radiotherapy Department was the first of many which eventually paved the way to the employment of the first HPS for radiotherapy but even then, the post was funded by a charity rather than the hospital for the first three years.

This pioneering time was often quite exhausting and remained a challenge for each subsequent HPS appointed to a new area of the hospital as the benefits of play were gaining recognition. When we expanded the play service fully into radiotherapy, most of the local staff had no sense of what the HPS was there to do (see Figure 1.2). The same thing happened with the first HPS in the Dental Hospital and in the Emergency Department. Explaining and, to some extent, justifying our existence required patience and tact, so it was extraordinarily satisfying when you won a 'convert', and the nurse, doctor or radiographer came to you asking for help with a child, *before* he or she became so distressed that you were their 'last chance'.

If staff involved me early, I could prepare the child for whatever procedure was to happen and significantly reduce the potential for distress and delay, so the 'conversion' benefitted both the child and the healthcare professional. Part of this education took place via the visible presence I had on the ward, in the shape of the playroom itself, and the playboxes in each treatment room, and also through my active participation in ward rounds and handovers. I am very grateful to the paediatrician in charge of the ward at the second hospital where I worked, who

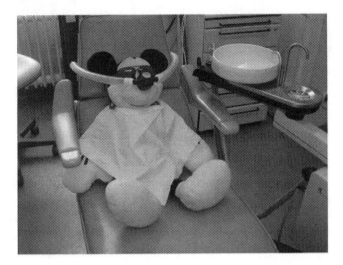

FIGURE 1.2 Mickey at the Dentist.

on the weekly 'Psychosocial' ward rounds would turn to me and say, "So Judy, what do you think?" as each child was discussed. Inviting me to share in this way meant I could no longer play the "I'm only a play specialist" card as I was being expected to contribute in the same way as every other health professional. It ensured that I had to rapidly formulate and articulate my assessments and observations of the child and family in as brief and professional manner as possible and it was a brilliant education for me, despite being terrifying at the time.

There were several other factors which contributed to my evolution towards being a healthcare professional who no longer introduced herself as "just the play specialist", as if my role was of lesser status than others. The first was the direct experience I gained from witnessing the outcomes of my play-based interventions for the child and the family. This taught me how powerful a child–centred approach is on all those involved and ensured my determination and advocacy remained strong. It also meant that even without role models to learn from, I would continue to improve and refine my approach.

Another key factor was learning about the need to speak in the language of the hospital rather than in the language of the playroom. To influence upwards and outwards, I developed ways to collect meaningful data about play activity and its changes over time. Numerical data gave substance to the concept of play and meant I was able to tell the story of the growing numbers of children using play facilities in each department and receiving specialist interventions. A transformational moment came when I was able to share data that proved the preparation through play of young children requiring radiotherapy led to significant cost savings as far fewer children needed to be admitted for a general anaesthetic to ensure they lay still for treatment. Reducing the number of general anaesthetics from 30 sessions to 0 for a course of radiotherapy was enormously beneficial to the child's health and well-being, but the motivation to eventually support the play service was driven by financial savings rather than child-centred care and safety.

This may seem surprising but the status of children in society was very different in the late 1980s and early 1990s, and the lack of interest in child-centred care and the associated low standing of the HPS role should be seen within this wider context. The UN Convention on the Rights of the Child was only ratified in the UK in 1991, and many jobs associated with children were routinely low paid and low in status. The caring and patient experience elements of healthcare were also relatively undervalued within the medical hierarchy. As children's rights have been recognised and their significance in society as consumers has changed, there has been a corresponding shift in understanding of their needs within the healthcare setting.

As well as educating others about the child's need for play to mitigate harm, I was also having to learn for myself how to work with the adults involved, both the staff on the ward and the parents of the children. Having not arrived on the ward via the traditional routes of medical or nursing school with many years as a junior doctor or student nurse, I had not been educated into the many implicit rules for behaviour. This sometimes resulted in getting told off by the Ward Sister. For example, I called the operating theatre which was waiting for five-year-old Jack and asked for the surgeon to come and reassure the child that he would only be taking out his tonsils and nothing else. At the time the child was hiding under the bed on the ward and had told me what he was scared of, so I knew that a chat with the surgeon would help. Thankfully, the surgeon came, sat on the floor next to the bed and provided Jack with the guarantee he needed and the operation went ahead smoothly. However, the ward Sister told me, "You can't just call the surgeon like that. You must come to me first".

One of the biggest challenges of working with parents was in getting them to trust that being honest with children was beneficial in the short and long term. Parents were happy for children to spend time in the playroom, but when inviting them to share with me what their child understood about an upcoming procedure, or their reason for admission, it was common to be told "she doesn't know anything" or "I don't want him to be told: it will only worry him". This denial of the reality that children will certainly know *something* is happening, and will *already* be worrying at some level of their consciousness, had to be addressed carefully. I had to learn to get the right balance between respecting the parental authority to know what is best for their child and educating them in the needs and rights of the child to have age appropriate information and the opportunity to develop coping strategies.

To help me deal with the steep learning curve I encountered as a young HPS, I wrote a reflective diary on a regular basis. Seeing the written words describing my work back at me helped me to make sense of it all. I was also helped by the ward's child psychotherapist, who gave me a language with which to articulate the things I observed, and a psychoanalytic framework within which to understand the child's behaviour. This gave flesh to the Piagetian developmental concepts which underpin hospital play specialism. I began to see that a child's play could have other meanings hidden in it. For example, I learned that for seven-year-old

Tim, with cancer and nursed in an isolation cubicle for many weeks during a long neutropenic phase, his frequent play with puppets and action men who were running free, climbing trees and fighting together helped him stay in touch with his normal 'healthy' self. Understanding these things meant I could explore with Tim some of the frustrations of being isolated from the outside world.

Sitting on my desk today is a small Royal Doulton china pot given to me by a patient's mother. She wanted to express her thanks for the care I had given to her daughter Dawn, who was treated for bone cancer. It was not unusual for any of us to receive a gift from parents who were grateful for the care given through the gruelling year-long treatment but this was exceptional. It arrived **three** years after Dawn had finished her chemotherapy and surgery. The note that came with the present from Mrs Hughes said that she had only recently understood from Dawn's reflections on her time on the ward, how important the time spent playing, talking and learning with me in the ward playroom had been. Mrs Hughes wanted to acknowledge how I had helped Dawn develop some healthy approaches to cope well during all the difficulties she encountered and how this had meant she had adjusted successfully to life back at school after treatment finished. This small gift and its message illustrate a valuable point: it can take a long time for the benefits of our work to be fully realised. It helps to be absolutely clear on what your purpose in any given situation is, even if others are not. Be guided by your professional values and ensure you learn from the experiences you have every day (see Figure 1.3).

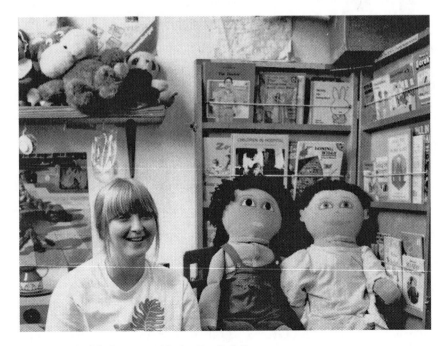

FIGURE 1.3 Judy's Corner, with the Zaadi dolls.

2

HOSPITAL: STILL A DEPRIVED ENVIRONMENT FOR CHILDREN?

Revisiting the case for hospital play

Cath Hubbuck – Senior Health Play Specialist

Joanne Cross – Senior Health Play Specialist

In 1989, Save the Children Fund (SCF) published a report which examined the impact of the experience of hospitalisation on children. The report also contained an evaluation of the impact of the hospital play schemes they were funding in hospitals at that time around the UK.

'Hospital: A Deprived Environment for Children?' – like the Platt Report released 30 years before it – clearly acknowledged that the hospital was a place where children were likely to experience stress and discomfort and, as a result, would struggle emotionally, socially and psychologically at the time and potentially after a hospital admission. It also stated that children in hospital have a particular 'special need for play', acknowledging therapeutic as well as developmental benefits of play for sick children. Lastly, the report placed an emphasis on the understanding that play should be provided by trained members of staff – health play specialists. As such, this report now represents part of the foundation for play provision in hospital today. It was an important document in the history and development of the health play specialist's role as we know it today.

In this chapter, we examine this document in context and the practical and legislative changes that have taken place affecting hospital play teams in the intervening years. We also reconsider the question it raised in 1989 of whether hospitals are still a 'deprived environment' for children (Figure 2.1).

The 1989 Save the Children report – the context and the impact

The SCF report was, first and foremost, a review of Save the Children funded hospital play provision for children in the UK. Additionally, having reviewed its current activity, it introduced a clear and specific rationale for the benefits of organised play services in hospital, warning of the risks to children's well-being

DOI: 10.4324/9781003255444-4

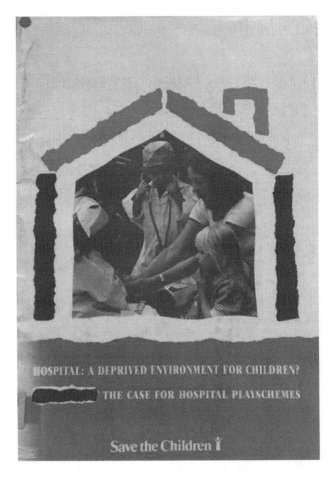

FIGURE 2.1 SCF report.

and development in the event of severe illness or injury and urging healthcare authorities who had not yet engaged in the cause to reconsider their provision for children.

This report came some 30 years after the Platt Report (Ministry of Health, 1959) and the groundbreaking late-1950s work of James and Joyce Robertson. The Robertsons were pioneering researchers who worked alongside the psychologist John Bowlby at the Tavistock Institute in London. The work of the institute at that time was focussed on "the loss of maternal care in the early years" (Robertson, 1970, p. ix). Through their work, the Robertsons developed a particular interest in the experiences of young children in hospital. In combination – but independent of each other – these two bodies of work had exposed the need for a change of approach to the ways that children received care when they were sick, by demonstrating the damaging impact on them of separation from their parents, the familiarity of home and usual childhood routines.

In the period that followed, some changes were clear and immediate. The training for and delivery of paediatric nursing and medical care underwent specific adjustments; accommodation was made for parents on hospital wards; and over time the expectation grew that, in the vast majority of cases, a parent would be resident with their child throughout their admission, as is the case today (Department of Health, 2003). The importance of and consideration for children's activities of daily living whilst in hospital also followed, and there was steady growth and development in the organisation of and specific employment for the delivery of play services for children in hospitals. Initially, after the release of the Platt Report, these were set up as individual 'playschemes' run by volunteers. However, in 1963 the first paid member of play staff – a play leader called Gabi Marston – was employed using funds from SCF at the Brook Hospital in South London (Marston, 2013).

Having achieved this milestone, campaigners for change in the provision of children's play in hospital recognised the need for a formalisation of specific training for play practitioners and the introduction of a professional job title duly followed. 'Hospital Play Specialist' (HPS) became recognised after the first training course was launched specifically for this role at Chiswick College in London in 1973.

Despite steady progress in establishing the profession of HPS in paediatric settings throughout the 1970s and 1980s, evidence gathered by the Save the Children and Play in Hospital Liaison Committee and presented in 1987 demonstrated that only 36% of children's wards in the UK had a 'playworker' in employment (Belson, 1987) – an increase from 14% ten years earlier. This was still a 'disturbingly low' statistic and healthcare providers were challenged that:

> If the hospital is to care for the whole child, physically, mentally and emotionally, it must provide suitable play facilities supervised by a trained member of staff as an integral part of the treatment plan.
>
> *Belson (1987, p. 16)*

In the same decade, the SCF – a prominent organisation, known for their humanitarian efforts in war-torn countries and situations of crisis, stated that their funding decisions concentrated on supporting children and families who experience the worst effects of deprivation. This statement, made in the introduction to the report, clearly indicated that the work of SCF included children, wherever they were in the world, with serious health problems and those in hospital.

The SCF report that is our focus in this chapter was released following many years of work by the Play in Hospital Liaison Committee who surveyed and presented the impact of the work of HPSs already employed and making a difference within children's healthcare. The intention of the committee by releasing the report was:

> to illustrate to those hospitals who have not yet recognised the need, the importance, for children and parents, of including a play specialist in the paediatric team.
>
> *Save the Children Fund (1989, n.pag.)*

It set out to present a theoretical understanding of play and the specific benefits of play for children whose development becomes disrupted by a period of illness and hospitalisation. The report aimed to be evidence-based, drawing predominantly from the practical experience of HPSs. It also raised a fundamental question of whether, despite advances in paediatric medicine and nursing approaches, places of healthcare could still be the cause of risk or disruption to the well-being of children, depriving them of the things fundamentally needed to develop and be content.

Ultimately, the SCF report concluded unequivocally that "children in hospital need play provision" (SCF, 1989, p. 30) and that this should be a matter of urgency to be addressed by local health authorities and the healthcare professionals charged with advising them. The belief in the importance of play within the care of sick children in hospital, and the need to value and purposefully employ qualified play specialists within paediatric multidisciplinary teams (MDTs), to ensure the provision of play happens lies at the heart of the report. Key statements also made were that "there is clearly still much to be done" in terms of recognising the importance of play for sick children (SCF, 1989, n.pag.) and also that matters around the standardisation of team structure and organisation (including pay and salary scales) were in progress but "not yet resolved" (p. 33).

Today's health play staff, therefore owes a lot to the SCF report. At the time of its release it brought about significant positive changes to the HPS profession. Thirty years on, however, we work in an ever-changing and developing health service, one that strives to be effective, efficient and for many can be life-saving, but one that is often also beset by problems and crises presented by funding and staffing, most recently by the extraordinary circumstances borne of the COVID-19 global pandemic.

Now, as we consider the provision of play for the next generation of children in hospitals, what do we see? Has there been progress in the role and work of hospital play staff? Has this progress been sustained? How have things changed for children in hospital?

Is hospital still 'a deprived environment for children'?

Legislative influences in children's healthcare and their impact on the work of HPSs

There have been many changes to the organisation and delivery of children's healthcare and how this is experienced by children, young people and their families. Immediately after the SCF report, two key documents were released that answered its call to action.

The first, in 1990, a document called *Quality Management for Children: Play in Hospital* (Hogg, 1990) was perhaps the most direct response. This comprised a set of guidelines for District Health Authorities dealing directly with how to assess the need for play within a variety of healthcare settings. The 1989 SCF report had not given a choice to healthcare providers but rather having made clear that organised, funded play provision in hospital was an expectation and essential for children and families. Thereafter it contained a set of guidelines for providers giving a detailed rationale for the value of play in particular hospital settings. This went beyond inpatient wards and included outpatient and accident and emergency departments. It then presented a checklist of what such provision should include in order to provide the highest quality for children. As such it could be used as a benchmarking tool by service providers and, in light of this, was well received by hospital play specialists and their employers at the time. 'The Green Book' – as Hogg's *Quality Management* document was informally known – was in use well into the late 1990s and early 2000s and set the foundations of many hospital play teams formed in that time.

This document is also significant to the profession because it was the first document that gave a recommendation on the number of trained HPSs that should be employed in paediatric settings. At this time a Department of Health 'Expert Group on Play' had recommended a level of staffing of one HPS for each ward or outpatients area. Furthermore, the group had considered what the 'optimum ratio' should be on an acute ward and, from this, the *Quality Management* report recommended a ratio of one play specialist to every ten patients (Hogg, 1990, p. 9). This was a powerful development for HPSs who now had a ratio for good practice and a figure to guide applications for both theoretical support and funding from local health boards. The precision of this recommended ratio was later lost in the 2003 National Service Framework for Children (NSF) legislation – a change that arguably, over time, has significantly impacted hospital play staff.

In 1991, The Department of Health published an updated policy document entitled *Welfare of Children and Young People in Hospital* which referenced both the SCF report and the *Quality Management* document. Here the statement was made that "play is essential" (Department of Health, 1991, p. 18) particularly for children in hospital, and the employment of play specialists as being central to the provision of play in healthcare settings was fully promoted. This document gave a detailed outline of the role of the HPS and stands as the first official government document to present them as professionals in their own right who should be present within modern paediatric MDTs.

Through to the turn of the last century, these pieces of legislation stood as the guidance on play provision in hospitals. In 2003 new guidance brought changes, the impact of which would be unexpectedly significant. TheNSF was released following investigations into the high-profile death of Victoria Climbie in 2001. This new legislation acknowledged that hospitals presented children and their families with "a daunting experience" and laid out guidance for the delivery of care that was "genuinely child-centred" (Department of Health, 2003, p. 1). The NSF legislation highlighted – and sought to significantly improve – the ways members of staff work together for the best possible care and outcomes for sick children. At the time of writing, it remains in place as the key guidance for paediatric healthcare within the National Health Service (NHS).

The real impact of the National Service Framework for Children

Within the NSF, HPSs are acknowledged to be key, established professionals working within the modern health service. They are mentioned in relation to normalising play and its benefits for children coming into hospital (p. 14), their role in preparing children for surgical or other invasive procedures (pp. 17, 29) and in the reduction of pain, distress or anxiety (p. 27). In many ways, the NSF was a key document for HPSs, setting out a position that placed play provision at the centre of children's hospital experiences. However, critical consideration of the NSF shows that it lacks the specified recommendations that were made in the earlier documents – recommendations that gave clear instructions on staffing ratios and the importance of their placement in particular areas of the hospital.

The NSF states that "all children staying in hospital should have daily access to a play specialist" (Department of Health, 2003, p. 15) – a powerful, but very broad statement and one lacking discussion or guidance about how teams should be organised or the ratio of patients, beds or paediatric units to play staff. While the positive and complimentary tone of the NSF seemed initially to be a great encouragement to the profession and an endorsement of the role of the HPS, the ambiguity of the outworking of playwork in hospital has – we would suggest – had significant implications for HPS practice in the intervening years. It has specifically made it challenging, for example, to appeal for increases in staff, since managers reviewing paediatric services could see a HPS in post and argue they are meeting the recommendation that all inpatients have 'daily access' to them alone. This fails to account for the HPS's workload, the number of children seen in inpatient wards, outpatient departments, ambulatory day care and emergency departments across a single hospital setting.

It is still not unheard of to find one HPS covering all these areas in a given setting, with no legislative support to meet any appeal for more staff. Crucially, this legislation has added to the debate over the value of play staff to hospitalised children, with several authors warning of the danger that they might be thought an expensive luxury that the healthcare can ill afford (Webster, 2000; Kennedy, 2010; Tonkin, 2014). Where expanded and expanding multi-level play teams exist in hospitals today, it is a testament to the effort of play staff themselves promoting their scope of work and managers recognising the need for more staff. Ultimately, this progress, where evident, has happened despite the content of the NSF not because of it.

Further legislative and constructive documents exist that have continued to embed the HPS within MDTs and to advocate for the impact and scope of their work. In 2010 the Kennedy Report (2010), commissioned by the government after the death of 'Baby P', raised an alarm that HPSs should be considered to be 'endangered' within the modern health service due to financial pressures and lack of recognition for their worth. Other documents continue to promote the benefits of play services (NICE, 2021) and, in some cases, the expectation that they will be running over seven days and accessible across all areas of the hospital (Shribman, 2014), without necessarily acknowledging that such services require ongoing investment in training and employing more members of staff. The ripples of the loss of HPS ratio specifications in the NSF are wide and considerable.

Progress and developments in the scope of the HPS's work – and challenges, too

Clearly in the 30 years since the SCF report, the medical and healthcare fields caring for children in hospitals have changed, progressed, improved and developed significantly. Medications and treatments have become much more sophisticated and advanced and in some disciplines, the approach to treating children's illness is almost unrecognisable. Continuous advances and research into the care of children with cancer and leukaemia, for example, mean the course of children's treatment has changed significantly and the survival rate for children with an oncology or haematology diagnosis is now more than 80%. In 1970, only three out of ten children with cancer were expected to survive their illness (Childhood Cancer and Leukaemia Group, 2017).

Changes and guidance relating to the care of babies, children and young people in hospitals and other healthcare settings have also developed. These have – in the main – consolidated a broad view that the care of children is important and should be both distinct in its approach and prioritised by everyone, from politicians and funding bodies to all those employed in healthcare settings for children.

In line with this progression, there is no doubt that the approach and hands-on work of HPSs have also developed to meet the needs of changing services. Hospitals now routinely employ HPSs to be based in speciality areas only, including oncology, general medicine, emergency departments and surgical or orthopaedic wards. There are also HPSs who work exclusively in MRI, imaging or radiotherapy departments helping children and young people to go through intensive treatment without sedation or anaesthetic. HPSs are also employed in hospices to provide specialised palliative care, and in the community, seeing children in their own homes and providing therapeutic spaces to prepare for hospital experiences. The question is do HPSs get the specialist training required to fully prepare and support the patients in their care or do they learn on their feet? Where is the education, supervision and support for HPSs venturing into new territories?

A major difficulty faced by today's HPSs – we observe – is that while their role is upheld by NHS providers and a set of standards for professional practice exists (HPSET, 2019), the very practical outworking of their scope of work is not clearly defined or standardised. In the years since 1989, despite several attempts, HPSs have not been able to achieve the status of being an Allied Health Professional. This has been due to a number of administrative barriers, but this achievement could have brought greater clarity and standardisation to the profession and maybe it could have contributed to settling the 'matters' described in the conclusion of the SCF report.

Instead, play services today are often stretched due to staffing costs, and there is little or no provision to backfill staff if they are sick or on maternity leave. Meanwhile, HPSs find themselves expanding their practice to respond to the complex needs of children and young people in hospital, but without the acknowledgment by managers or provision for the extra time this work might take. The role is often seen as fun and frivolous, while not always acknowledging the targeted and complex work that HPSs are doing with children through play.

The lack of a 'professional status' has an impact on the practice of HPSs. The way play teams are structured continues to vary significantly between healthcare trusts, with each hospital using their own somewhat 'organic' model of what a play service looks like. This brings with it its own standards and expectations of how the service will run from its management structure to how play is resourced and delivered in each area. Recruitment processes, play policies, documentation and play programmes are all differently developed within individual healthcare trusts meaning there is not a single, transferable template for services to universally use. The result feels like a somewhat fragmented profession. The sense of what 'Best Practice' looks like in each hospital or healthcare trust looks and feels different and is bound by such variable factors as funding, management and staff expectations. The experience for children receiving hospital care arguably is variable too. As a profession, without centralised guidance or consultation, HPSs cannot guarantee every child will be in receipt of the same quality of care and equitable attention from play services in one setting as they will be in another.

PANDEMIC = PLAY PARALYSIS?

The pandemic was an unprecedented and extraordinary event in human history.

As a profession health play staff definitely had to learn – and learn fast! – on the job. There was little or no guidance on the issues faced by play staff, and most decisions on how to run a daily play service in these new and daunting circumstances were made locally. Some trusts allowed play specialists to support patients with COVID-19 whilst wearing full personal protective equipment (PPE), whereas other trusts would only allow play specialists to work in 'green' (clean and Covid-free) areas. Once again play teams across the UK were doing things slightly differently and had no central source of information to refer to or draw upon.

The COVID-19 pandemic had a significant impact on hospital play service provision. At the time of writing, more than two and a half years beyond the earliest restrictions, many play teams are still only able to offer reduced play activities. Throughout the pandemic a major part of the role of play teams has been cleaning, ensuring that resources are cleaned and sterilised after each use. This has been incredibly time-consuming and has impacted on the available play provision for patients. For the first year of the pandemic, at least, resources and activities had to be limited to disposable single use craft packs.

Crucially, in March 2020, hospital playrooms – which, in most children's wards, had been open-access spaces for children and young people – were immediately closed. By mid-2022 some of these playrooms had reopened but with a changed set-up. On some wards, children can access the playroom, but just on their own with a parent or play assistant, rather than mixing freely with other patients of their own age. Some play teams lost their play spaces altogether and – in some healthcare trusts – it seems unlikely these will be returned. Playrooms remain closed and some have even been permanently repurposed to allow for staff breakout spaces or offices.

The pandemic has shown how vulnerable children are in hospital when their access to play – especially their ability to freely access play spaces – becomes extremely limited. In 2014, Alison Tonkin observed that for children in hospital the right to play has an even greater importance than for most children, but that those children will need extra or specific help to fulfil that right (Tonkin, 2014, p. 21). That specific help predominantly comes directly from hospital play staff who understand and can assess the urgency of their need. When the pandemic began, the ability of play staff to practice as they always had was radically affected and even where there has been creative adaptation, at the time of writing play practice in hospitals has largely still not fully recovered.

As much as the pandemic has shown the vulnerability of children in hospital when play provision is suddenly and dramatically impacted, it has also shone a light on the vulnerability of play services in hospital themselves.

Ultimately, the loss of play spaces and social contact through play and the limits placed on play staff is a loss that has affected children and young people for whom the playroom was a haven from the relentlessness of hospital treatment.

Does this make for a deprived environment? We believe it does.

So, is hospital still 'a deprived environment for children'?

The use of the word 'deprivation' in the original 1989 SCF report is perhaps the feature that was so significant on its release. As a society that claims to value children and the well-being of children, almost to the exclusion of all else, to consider a place of care to also be a place of deprivation was both shocking and stark. Perhaps it still is now? After all, it is clear that the risks of distress and discomfort are high for children in hospital (Lansdown, 1996; Walker, 2006; Hubbuck, 2009; Carter and Simons, 2014; Tonkin, 2014; NICE, 2021; Perez-Duarte, 2022).

Whenever a child becomes separated from the things that matter to them and admitted to hospital, all the familiarity and feelings of safety associated with those things will potentially be lost, even if only temporarily. In the 1950s, the Robertsons presented the case that children's bonds of attachment to their mothers were disrupted, even damaged, by time spent in hospital (Robertson, 1970). We now understand attachment in a more nuanced way, understanding that attachments – important relationships that foster a sense of safety and an understanding of self – extend well beyond mothers to include other important people, places, pets, significant items as well as more abstract things such as regular routines (Conkbayir and Pascal, 2014). Separated from these things, children in hospital also stand to encounter uncomfortable interventions and physical restrictions including the freedom to play.

This combination of factors means that, when they are in hospital, children are at a higher risk of both developmental disruption and the risk of emotional harm in both the short and the long term.

In the years since the SCF report, these risks have been highlighted by important national and international organisations including UNICEF (1989), Play England (2008), Play Scotland (2011) and Brown (2013 – for Play Wales). In 2014 the International Play Association (IPA) produced an agreed definition of 'play deprivation'. This definition was part of a broader 'Declaration on the Importance of Play' and acknowledged that "not playing deprives children of experiences that are regarded as developmentally essential" (IPA, 2014, p. 3). A later document also released by the IPA (2017) went on to recognise the importance of children's ability to have access to play in situations of crisis and included both ill-health and displacement in its criteria for the consideration of what constitutes 'a crisis'. In addition to this, a broad global understanding of trauma and the effects of 'toxic stress' has developed and deepened in many areas of academic expertise and practical hands-on health and social care (Nelson et al., 2020).

In conclusion ...

It was important to acknowledge the uncomfortable incongruence that was presented by SCF in their report in 1989 – that a place of care could also be neglectful and therefore, in some way, uncaring. That incongruence still feels alarming today. However, the answer to the question posed by SCF all those years ago is that yes, without doubt, hospital is still a deprived environment for children – **and it probably always will be.**

The hospital environment carries high risks from a multitude of factors for children and young people. To ensure the continuation of the provision of play – rich, meaningful, informative and supportive play – even in times of great social, political or global upheaval, is also to ensure the provision of emotional, social and psychological 'buffers' for the youngest patients within our national health services.

References

Belson, P (1987) A Plea for Play. *Nursing Times* 83 (26) pp. 16–17

Brown, F. (2013) *Play Deprivation: Impact, Consequences and the Potential of Playwork.* [Online] Available from: <https://issuu.com/playwales/docs/play_deprivation_impact_consequence> [Accessed 17 June 2022]

Carter, B. and Simons, J. (2014) *Stories of Children's Pain*. London: Sage

Childhood Cancer and Leukaemia Group (2017) *Annual Review 2017*. [Online] Available from: <https://www.cclg.org.uk/write/MediaUploads/About%20CCLG/Annual%20reviews/CCLG_Annual_Review_2017_Web_Final.pdf> [Accessed 15 March 2022]

Cole-Hamilton, I. and Play Scotland (2011) *Getting It Right for Play. Children's Play in Scotland: The Policy Context*. Roslin Midlothian: Play Scotland

Conkbayir, M. and Pascal. C. (2014) *Early Childhood Theories and Contemporary Issues*. London: Bloomsbury

Department of Health (1991) *Welfare of Children and Young People in Hospital*. London: Department of Health

Department of Health (2003) *Getting the Right Start: National Service Framework for Children. Standards for Hospital Services*. London: Department of Health

Hogg, C. (1990) *Quality Management for Children: Play in Hospital*. London: Save the Children

HPSET (Health Play Specialist Education Trust) (2019) *Health Play Specialist Standards of Proficiency Professional Standards*. [Online] Available from: <https://hpset.org.uk/HPSET_ps.pdf> [Accessed 3 May 2022]

Hubbuck, C. (2009) *Play for Sick Children: Play Specialists in Hospital and Beyond*. London: Jessica Kingsley Publishers

International Play Association (IPA) (2014) *Declaration on the Importance of Play*. London. [Online] Available from: <http://ipaworld.org/wp-content/uploads/2015/05/IPA_Declaration-FINAL.pdf> [Accessed 17 June 2022]

International Play Association (IPA) (2017) *Access to Play for Children in Situations of Crisis. Play: Rights and Practice: A Toolkit for Staff, Managers and Policy Makers*. London: IPA

Kennedy, I. (2010) *Getting It Right for Children and Young People. Overcoming Cultural Barriers in the NHS so as to Meet Their Needs*. London: Department of Health

Lansdown, R. (1996) *Children in Hospital: A Guide for Parents and Carers*. Oxford: Oxford University Press

Marston, G. (2013) The Birth of Hospital Playschemes. *The Journal of the National Association of Health Play Specialists*. [Online] Available from: <https://www.nahps.org.uk/wp-content/uploads/2018/08/NAHPS-Journal-Spring-2013.pdf> [Accessed 2 July 2022]

Ministry of Health (1959) *The Welfare of Children in Hospital* (commonly known as *The Platt Report*). London: Ministry of Health

Nelson, C., Bhutta, Z., Burke Harris, N., Danese, A., and Samara, M. (2020) Adversity in Childhood is Linked to Mental and Physical Health Throughout Life. *BMJ* 2020 371 pp. m3048

NICE (2021) *Babies, Children's and Young People Experiences of Healthcare (NICE Guideline 204)*. National Institute for Clinical Excellence. [Online] Available from: <https://www.nice.org.uk/guidance/ng204/informationforpublic> [Accessed 1 July 2022]

Perez-Duarte, P (2022) How to Communicate with Children According to Health Play Specialists in the United Kingdom: A Qualitative Study. *Journal of Child Health Care*. [Online] Available from: <https://journals.sagepub.com/doi/pdf/10.1177/13674935221109113> [Accessed 20 June 2022]

Powell, S., and Wellard, I. (2008) *Policies and Play: the Impact of National Policies on Children's Opportunities for Play*. London: Play England

Robertson, J. (1970) *Young Children in Hospital*. 2nd ed. London: Tavistock

Save the Children Fund (SCF) (1989) *Hospital: A Deprived Environment for Children. The Case for Hospital Playschemes*. London: Save the Children Fund

Shribman, S. (2014) *Getting It Right for Children & Young People (Including Those Transitioning into Adult Services): A Report on CQC's New Approach to Inspection.* [Online] Available from: <https://www.cqc.org.uk/sites/default/files/20140331%20Dr%20Sheila%20Shribman%20report%20to%20CIOH%20re%20inspection%20of%20CYP%20services....pdf> [Accessed 2 July 2022]

Tonkin, A. (2014) *The Provision of Play in Health Service Delivery: Fulfilling Children's Rights under Article 31 of the United Nations Convention on the Rights of the Child. A Literature Review.* [Online] Available from: <https://www.england.nhs.uk/6cs/wp-content/uploads/sites/25/2015/03/nahps-full-report.pdf> [Accessed 18 May 2022]

Unicef (1989) *The United Nations Convention on the Rights of the Child.* [Online] Available from: <https://www.unicef.org.uk/wp-content/uploads/2016/08/unicef-convention-rights-child-uncrc.pdf> [Accessed 2 July 2022]

Walker, J. (2006) *Play for Health: Delivering and Auditing Quality in Hospital Play Services.* London: NAHPS

Webster, A. (2000) The Facilitating Role of the Play Specialist. *Paediatric Nursing* 12(7) pp. 24–27

3

IT PAYS TO PLAY!

How I discovered cost-effective play and the start of the MRI Awake List Project

Irene O'Donnell – NHS Hospital Trust lead for therapeutic play, recreation, and youth services

The National Health Service (NHS) is faced with continuous demands both financially and with capacity, never more so than during the past few years when we have experienced the COVID-19 pandemic. Due to this it has become increasingly challenging to provide care at the point of need in an efficient way that retains a positive patient and staff experience. Highlighting opportunities for decreasing costs and improving experience needs to be explored and encouraged. One innovative way of doing this is supporting children and young people (CYP) to have MRI scans awake, using play instead of general anaesthetic (GA) or sedation. But convincing colleagues or NHS managers who hold responsibility for budgets that investing in play can bring cost savings and improve capacity can be a challenge! It involves taking a risk that this will work and not cause more issues, such as wasted slots if the CYP cannot cooperate. The question is always: where is your evidence? The question is a valid one, as without evidence to prove the benefits or improvements it is often perceived as a 'nice to have' or luxury item in the shopping basket rather than an essential ingredient for all CYP in healthcare.

So, the question that faces us as Health Play Specialists (HPS) is, how do we convince people it really does pay to play?

Why play?

Play is a child's natural tool for learning about the world around them. It can bring valuable therapeutic benefits and feelings of calmness and well-being (Brown & Vaughan, 2009). According to the United Nations Convention on the Rights of the Child (UNCRC), all children have the right to access play and recreation wherever they are, including in healthcare. Play has the simple but important function of introducing something familiar to the often unfamiliar environment

DOI: 10.4324/9781003255444-5

of hospitals and gives the significant message to children that when attending hospitals with play available they are welcome and appreciated (Walker, 2006).

MRI scans

According to a recent article published in The Mail Online approximately 150,000 CYP per year in the UK require an MRI scan (Henderson, 2022). There are many challenges that face CYP when coming for an MRI, as the scanner is large and can feel somewhat intimidating. The MRI scanner can be very loud and will move frequently during the scan to get the images required. All this sensory input and fear of the unknown is the perfect recipe for an anxious and non-cooperative child who will be too scared to attempt to lie down and stay still. The missing ingredient in the recipe to improve this situation is play!

My journey of discovery, with it pays to play!

I first identified the need to support children to undertake MRI scans while awake in 2007 when I was working as a Senior HPS in a busy London Hospital Trust. This was following the development of new MRI techniques to assess iron load in patients. These techniques were being installed in MRI suites not suitable for general anaesthesia (unlike the standard ones used for MRI of the brain), a situation that presented a challenge to the medical team and the play specialist – me!

When presented with this challenge during a multidisciplinary team (MDT) discussion, I proposed using play to prepare the CYP for the scan and 'breath-holding' and plan a coping strategy with the CYP and their family to manage the scan with the child awake. It is fair to say there was doubt in the room! One of the CYP being proposed was three years old. How would a HPS be able to get them to stay still and hold their breath? I felt confident in both my ability to empower the child to do this and in their ability to succeed. Children are remarkable in their ability to cope with many things adults would not fare so well at. Following discussion and presenting information on the benefits of play for CYP in hospital, I persuaded a MDT to trust the idea and agree to implement this new pathway. The child in discussion had iron overload and needed a bone marrow transplant, so the scan was important. I went to the scanner for a visit, took some photos and talked to the radiographer so I could prepare the child with all the key information.

We had a talented technician who made a mini model scanner for us to use. We used a tape recording of the sound of the scanner to demonstrate this to the CYP (how things have evolved!). The child managed the scan well with everything we had prepared and practised. With the success of the first scan, I started to receive more requests for support with similar procedures. With my confidence growing in my ability to prepare CYP to manage without GA, and in the CYP's ability to cope once they knew what was happening, I began to challenge decisions appropriately in MDT discussions when CYP were booked to have scans or procedures with sedation or GA – why can we not prepare them through play instead?

The success had huge benefits for CYPs treatment, enabling MDTs to personalise treatment previously not possible. It significantly improved patient experiences, reduced hospitalisation time for the CYP and families, and improved resource use and efficiency and safety by avoiding pharmalogical interventions. All of this was possible with the power of play and the role of the HPS – maybe it does pay to play?!

The development of the MRI awake list at UCLH

University College London Hospital NHS Foundation Trust (UCLH) is one of the largest NHS trusts in the UK and comprises of ten hospitals providing first-class acute and specialist care (UCLH, 2022). UCLH is a leader in the use of play specialists to avoid GA and had a very established and successful model within their radiotherapy department supporting CYP to have radiotherapy treatment without GA since 2000.

Following my move to UCLH in 2011, I recognised that many CYP were being booked for MRI scans under GA or sedation and often heard challenges from my colleagues with bed capacity and waiting lists. I knew that using a HPS and play could help resolve this challenge and luckily for me I now had some evidence to strengthen the case for it pays to play!

Using the successful model in radiotherapy and my previous work with MRI T2★ as examples, I engaged proactively in discussions with colleagues who championed the concept of using play. I planned and implemented a trial post and service that we would audit, and from which we would collect data to provide evidence to measure the outcomes. The Band 6 HPS post began with a 9-month trial carried out by an established member of the team, seconded to support MRI for one day a week. During this time, the HPS supported 42 patients (aged 4–8 years of age), 38 of which were successful in having their MRI scan without GA. The HPS-supported paediatric 'awake' list was developed, reducing waiting times for MRI under GA by 24%. The HPS also sought feedback from the CYP and staff. A proposal for a permanent Imaging HPS was presented to senior management, resulting in a new Band 6 HPS post for 3.5 days a week (2 days in Imaging, 1.5 days in Nuclear Medicine) in 2015.

Since the post was established over 8 years ago at 3.5 days a week, the Imaging HPSs, kept data detailing the support and outcomes of patients having procedures both in the Imaging and Nuclear Medicine departments at UCLH. Together we submitted a successful bid in 2020 to demonstrate the need for the post to be extended from 0.7 to 1.2 WTE to meet the growing service needs. This was justified by the evidential data and literature we had gathered over the years of running the MRI 'awake' list, and which was used as part of a UCLH Imaging bid.

We co-designed an MRI Awake Pathway (above four years old, refer to HPS for play prep.) to formalise how the new system would work. This was then used as the new pathway for clinicians referring any CYP for an MRI scan.

The HPS provides developmentally appropriate support to CYP and their families for scanning procedures prior to, during, and after the scan. Often, this is with little warning and time for rapport building, so expert skill is required to build a therapeutic relationship. On other occasions, CYP are referred in advance, so the HPS has more time to liaise with the MDT and CYP to support them through the scan. The UCLH mini-MRI model (made by Ernie Palfi) is a valuable tool to help demonstrate to the CYP what the scan will involve, feel look, and sound like.

An MRI compatible DVD player has been another valuable piece of equipment to support CYP to manage the scan and with preparation from the HPS, use this as a focus activity to stay still during the scan (Figure 3.1).

When the post was created, it was among the first of its kind across the UK. Since then, it has been recognised for its good practice which has been shared with colleagues around the country. Other NHS Trusts have used the UCLH model, and now have successful Imaging HPS posts and MRI Awake lists. The Imaging HPS role/awake list was shortlisted for a British Medical Journal (BMJ) innovation award (2018), the UCLH Excellence Award (2019), and more recently, the post has been nominated and recognised for a Getting It Right First Time Award (2021).

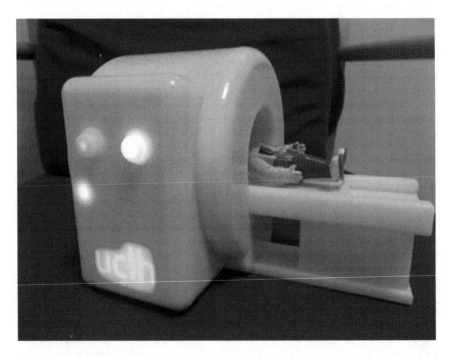

FIGURE 3.1 MRI scanner.

(A model MRI scanner complete with lights and noise created by Ernie Palfi, UCLH).

Following the success of the MRI Awake project, I was invited by the Royal College of Anaesthetists to join a discussion on the review of the NICE guidelines for CYP having sedation and GA. The concept of using the HPS's play preparation as an alternative option to sedation or GA was raised and acknowledged along with the involvement of the CYP in decision-making process (NICE, 2021).

Results

Vital to the success of the project was to have 'champions' and support from key colleagues to positively embrace the new way of working.

As the play services manager I had to build the case for a HPS in MRI and illustrate the benefits to the organisation in fiscal savings, increased efficiency, and patient experience that this could bring. The Consultant Paediatrician championed the pathway and modelling this with her colleagues was crucial to getting the team to adopt the new pathway and referral to the HPS for play rather than GA.

The lead Paediatric Radiographer was key in her role of identifying the patients suitable for awake MRI via requests coming into the imaging team and monitoring any children referred for GA that were over four years and had not been referred to the play specialist awake list.

MDT collaborative working has been at the heart of the success of this project and the benefits to patients and families have been vast:

- Reducing need for admission to hospital
- Avoiding the use of pharmaceutical interventions
- Reducing length of visit
- Reducing waiting times for appointments
- Improving patient experiences
- Building resilience in CYP to manage procedures

We currently have expanded the Awake List to facilitate up to ten CYP every Tuesday morning and more throughout the week as needed.

It pays to play: Getting It Right First Time (GIRFT)

University College London Hospitals NHS Foundation Trust has appointed a Band 6 HPS who now works with 95% of children needing an MRI. It has found that around nine children a week, who would previously have required a general anaesthetic for MRI, now receive an MRI without one. As well as benefiting the individual children, this also means that the time needed for these MRIs is reduced – freeing up additional imaging sessions.

Halliday et al. (2020, p. 24)

Conclusion

The HPS can facilitate opportunities to prepare CYP for procedures that would commonly involve the use of pharmacological interventions such as sedation/ GA as well as a hospital admission. Non-pharmacological techniques such as distraction and coping strategies, along with preparation and information sharing, have demonstrated:

- A decrease in anxiety experienced by CYP and their family
- Increased efficiency in services
- Decrease in time taken to do the procedure
- Reduced safety risks for patients (GA)
- Reduced waiting lists
- Reduced likelihood of a failed procedure
- An increase in building resilience and coping strategies for future procedures

Halliday et al. (2020)

As Jessie J once sang, "*It's not about the money, money, money…*" well sometimes in play it can be … it really does pays to play!

References

Brown, S. and Vaughan, C. (2009) *Play. How it Shapes the Brain, Opens the Imagination, and Invigorates the Soul.* New York: Penguin Group

Halliday, K., Maskell, G., Beeley, L. and Quick, E. (2020) *Radiology GIRFT Programme National Specialty Report.* [Online] Available from: <https://www.gettingitrightfirsttime. co.uk/wp-content/uploads/2020/11/GIRFT-radiology-report.pdf> [Accessed June 2022]

Henderson, C. (2022) *Lego Kit That Shows Kids What It's Like to Have an MRI – So the Real Thing Won't Be as Frightening.* [Online] The Mail Online. Available from: <https:// www.mailplus.co.uk/edition/health/medical-matters/170444/lego-kit-that-shows-kids-what-its-like-to-have-an-mri-so-the-real-thing-wont-be-as-frightening> [Accessed June 2022]

NICE (2021) *Shared Decision Making.* [Online] National Institute for Health and Care Excellence. Available from: <https://www.nice.org.uk/about/what-we-do/our-programmes/nice-guidance/nice-guidelines/shared-decision-making> [Accessed July 2022]

UCLH (2022) *University College London Hospitals NHS Foundation Trust.* [Online] Available from: < https://www.uclh.nhs.uk/> [Accessed 12 August 2022]

Walker, J. (2006) *Play for Health: Delivering and Auditing Quality in Hospital Play Services.* London: National Association of Hospital Play Staff

4

SUPPORT FOR SIBLINGS DURING THE MEDICAL JOURNEY

Charlotte Hamflett – Health Play Specialist

Just as the impact of acute ill-health, hospitalisation, or chronic illness may have lasting psychosocial consequences for children and their parents, the well-being of healthy siblings can also be affected by their brother or sister's medical journey.

It is not just extended stays in hospital or serious illness that impact siblings. A visit to Accident and Emergency or a short hospital admission can likewise affect a sibling's well-being. Siblings may retain unpleasant memories of watching a brother or sister's injury occur or seeing their sibling unwell or in distress. Additionally, they may harbour feelings of guilt that they were in some way responsible for their brother or sister's illness or injury.

In a school environment, I supported nine-year-old Remy whose baby sister was admitted to hospital with bronchiolitis. Usually a sociable child, he appeared uncharacteristically withdrawn and became tearful during lessons. When I sat with him, Remy described frightening memories of his sister struggling to breathe and how he hated thinking of his baby sister with her head in a box in hospital. He went on to say that he had found it hard to sleep the previous night because he could not stop worrying and missed his mother and sister.

I drew Remy a picture of the oxygen head box his father had told him about. He was relieved that it was made of clear plastic, not cardboard, and that his mum could still play with his sister while she breathed extra oxygen to make her feel better.

Remy seemed to relax as he drew a picture of his family, with vibrant colours for his dad to place next to his sister's cot. Although still worried, Remy subsequently appeared more himself and better able to focus on his work for the rest of the morning.

DOI: 10.4324/9781003255444-6

Figure 4.1 illustrates a wide range of factors that may impact the well-being of siblings of sick children (see next page).

Worryingly, White et al. (2017, p. 2) observed that siblings of children with chronic illnesses experience, "an elevated risk for psychological distress, poorer psychological functioning, engagement in fewer peer activities, and lower cognitive development scores". Although many children with well controlled chronic conditions remain well and require few medical interventions, routine outpatient appointments may trigger feelings of anxiety for siblings. Due to childcare constraints, or to help them feel involved, brothers and sisters are often brought along to after school appointments or treatments during school holidays. While the parent accompanies the patient, siblings may be left in the waiting room, or they sit in the corner of the treatment room and subsequently hear their sibling in distress.

The value of preparing, including, and reassuring siblings cannot be underestimated. I have worked with children of all ages, who have questioned "… What are they doing to my sister? Why are they hurting her?"

Some verbalised anger towards their sibling's illness and even towards practitioners caring for them, whereas others had misconceptions about their sibling's treatment. For example, six-year-old Jess told me "… Sammy screams when he has blood tests because he hates the nurse pealing back his skin to get the blood out".

Medical role play is a powerful tool in sibling support. By playing through procedures with siblings, play practitioners impart clarity and reassurance, thus, helping them to understand procedures in an age-appropriate, meaningful way, correcting misconceptions, desensitising them to medical equipment, and providing them with opportunities to ask questions.

Siblings of children with debilitating or harder to regulate conditions, such as osteogenesis imperfecta or severe epilepsy, are more likely to be impacted by their sibling's ill health than those whose siblings have well-controlled illnesses. Their sick brothers and sisters may experience frequent flare ups and require more health appointments, admissions, and interventions, resulting in repeated upheavals to routine and family life. They may also be acutely aware of the impact of stress and pressures on their parents, causing them to worry not just for their sick sibling but also for their family. In my experience as a play specialist, the cumulative impact of exposure to parental anxiety, coping with their own emotions and observing their brother or sister experience repeated trauma and admissions, can have a lasting effect on sibling well-being.

Reassuringly, Fleary and Heffer (2013) identified that, being a sibling to a chronically ill child also correlates to a high level of positive outcomes in adolescence, including "appreciation of life" (para. 19). They also suggest that cautiousness about health and maturity may act as protective variables, and characteristics such as empathy and compassion may benefit young people as they transition to adulthood and form lasting friendships and relationships.

Siblings may enter a hospital for the first time when visiting their sick brother or sister. Hospital visits can generate a range of emotions. They may be not only excited about seeing their sibling and the parent who has been resident with

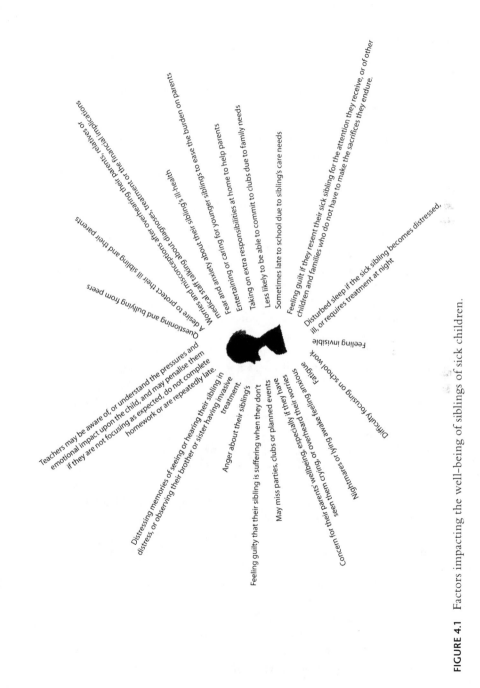

FIGURE 4.1 Factors impacting the well-being of siblings of sick children.

them but also anxious as to what they will see and hear in the hospital setting. They may resent having to miss activities such as football or dancing to visit or be envious of gifts and attention their sick sibling is receiving. Likewise, the patient may be apprehensive about having visitors. In my experience, sick children and young people sometimes become withdrawn when visitors arrive. This often reflects a desire to hide their experiences and emotions, or feelings of embarrassment and shame about changes to their bodies such as burns, scars, or hair loss.

On busy wards, siblings may feel they are in the way or be reprimanded by their parents or staff for being a nuisance. This can yield feelings of rejection. By spending time with siblings in the playroom, or interacting with them at the bedside, play staff have an influential role in making siblings feel welcome in the hospital environment. More than merely keeping them occupied whilst their parents spend time with their unwell sibling or meet with the medical team, play practitioners can communicate that they are important too.

The following story of Theo demonstrates how play can change a child's understanding and showcases the power of age-appropriate explanations that can reframe scary and alien looking medical equipment.

Three-year-old Theo arrived with his aunt to see his mother and meet his brother, Max, in the Neonatal Intensive Care Unit (NICU). He ran towards his mother who was sat by Max's incubator. She beamed as she saw Theo, but grimaced, clearly in pain, as he jumped up to her to give her a hug. She cuddled and interacted playfully with him.

After a few minutes, his aunt lifted Theo so he could see his brother. Max, who was delivered at 29 weeks, was hooked up to monitors, had a nasal-gastric tube and sported a peripheral cannular. Theo looked enquiringly at his mother, asking "but where's my baby?" He fidgeted, seemingly wanting to get down, and ran out of the room when the incubator started bleeping.

The mother wept. While her sister comforted her, I followed Theo to the family room. Theo sat holding a car. I too picked up a car and we raced our cars across the floor for a few minutes. I asked him if he would like to choose three cars to show Mummy.

Once the family had settled, looking at the cars together, I approached his mother to ask if I might show Theo Max's 'spaceship-cot'. I explained that NICU could be a strange, intimidating environment for a young child and that although Theo had been told his newborn brother was very tiny, his expectation of Max may be more like the babies he saw at nursery. It was discussed that Theo might understand more if information was likened to concepts he could imagine or had experience of.

Subsequently, his mother explained to Theo that Max had been so excited to meet him that he had come out of her tummy a bit early. Because he was so tiny, the doctors and nurses were looking after him and he would be having sleepovers at the hospital with the other tiny babies until he got a bit bigger. I took my cue from the mother, and whilst kneeling on the floor with Theo, explained that Max had his own special spaceship cot. It was a bit noisy and had lights that told the nurses how Max was feeling.

As we walked around the incubator with his aunt, I stated that the buttons on the side made the spaceship-cot warm and cosy. I also told Theo that tiny babies need to sleep a lot. So that they didn't have to keep waking Max up to check on him or give him his milk, the doctors and nurses had:

- Put special stickers on his chest that told them how he was feeling
- Given him a special straw in his nose to drink his milk through
- Put a super special straw on his arm to give him medicine to help him grow big and strong

His aunt lifted Theo again. He looked with fascination at his brother, who wriggled. Theo giggled and announced. "Mummy, he moved!"

As the family played in the family room, I gathered a bandage and a neonatal heart monitoring sticker so Theo could play doctors and nurses at home and take them to 'show and tell' at nursery.

Play and activities involving the whole family are key to facilitating normality and fun in a potentially threatening medical environment, lessening emotional barriers and creating positive memories, making siblings feel they are a part of their brother or sister's medical journey.

To maintain their ill sibling's links with home and school and to give them a role, brothers and sisters may be tasked with making videos of family pets or collecting messages from friends and teachers. In turn they may be kept informed with video diaries from their brother or sister and their resident parent.

Emotional support for siblings is paramount if a brother or sister's condition is life changing or life threatening. Smardakiewicz et al. (2004, p. 323) stated:

> The presence of childhood cancer threatens the balance of the entire family. Perhaps the most profoundly affected are the healthy siblings, who experience significant psychological distress at home as well as school. They suffer from a lack of knowledge about their brother or sister's disease, feelings of abandonment, anger, resentment, sadness, and guilt.

Fundamental to supporting siblings at this difficult time is the empowerment of their parents. Helping them to acknowledge and outpour their own feelings, and to understand how their 'healthy' children may be feeling, could be the first step in enabling them to find the words and the courage to talk to their children about their sibling's illness. According to Rozdilsky (2005), distraught parents may not have the insight to identify the needs of their well children, not know how to explain the situation or even realise that well siblings benefit from being with their ill sister or brother.

Having a member of the healthcare team to explain the situation to siblings, or to encourage the siblings to express their thoughts and emotions to someone

---

Rafiq and his 14-year-old sister Alima had cystic fibrosis. Over several years, I built a rapport with them both during clinic appointments and short admissions.

When Alima was admitted to the High Dependency Unit, awaiting a transplant, their mother was resident. Rafiq and their other siblings were staying with grandparents. Rafiq visited as often as possible and sat with his sister, chatting to try and make her smile, or watching movies with her. One afternoon, I challenged him to a game of table football while Alima was having a cannula inserted. Part way through the game he hung his head low and started twiddling one of the handles. When I acknowledged that he seemed troubled, Rafiq burst into tears.

I made him tea and toast in the teenage sitting room. Sobbing, Rafiq queried:

"What if she dies? Is this going to happen to me?"

As we sat, Rafiq also expressed fears about the emotional impact Alima's deterioration was having on their mother and one of his other siblings. He had not told anyone about his thoughts and feelings because he hated thinking about what might happen and didn't want to burden anyone

---

outside the family, can be a relief to parents and children. Art, role play, and age-appropriate games may provide openings to start such conversations, as illustrated by the story of 12-year-old Rafiq.

Sensitive preparation, therapeutic art, and normalising play are valuable in helping children and young people cope with their sibling's acute ill health and prognosis. Even during end-of-life care, play can bring comfort and moments of joy to the sick child and their family. Engaging gently with their loved one in sensory activities, decorating their brother or sister's room and sharing favourite music and films may give siblings and their parents a sense that they are doing something meaningful and enable them to build precious memories and familiarity when reality feels too much to bear.

In closing, normalising play and play interventions can be greatly beneficial when supporting the siblings of sick children. Play practitioners are skilled at identifying siblings who are in difficulty and in guiding them to express and cope with their experiences and emotions while advocating for the needs of siblings and families to the rest of the multidisciplinary team.

References

Fleary, S., and Heffer, R. (2013) Impact of Growing up with a Chronically Ill Sibling on Well Siblings' Late Adolescent Functioning, *ISRN Family Medicine* 2013 [Online] Available from: <https://www.ncbi.nlm.nih.gov/pmc/articles/PMC4041246/> [Accessed 17 June 2022]

Rozdilsky, J.R. (2005) Enhancing Sibling Presence in Pediatric ICU, *Critical Care Nursing Clinics of North America* 17 (4), p. 451

Smardakiewicz, M., Krukowska, E., and Kowalczyk, J. (2004) Healthy Siblings of Children with Cancer. The Model of Psychosocial Care, *Medycyna Wieku Rozwojowego* 8 (2) (part 1), pp. 323–332, cited in English at PubMed [Online] Available from: <https://pubmed.ncbi.nlm.nih.gov/15738609/> [Accessed 17 June 2022]

White, T., Hendershot, K., Dixon, M., Pelletier, W., Haight, A., Stegenga, K., Alderfer, M., Cox, L., Switchenko, J., Hinds, P., and Pentz, R. (2017) Family Strategies to Support Siblings of Hematopoietic Stem Cell Transplant Patients, *Pediatrics* 139 (2) [Online] Available from: <https://publications.aap.org/pediatrics/article-abstract/139/2/e20161057/60302> [Accessed 17 June 2022]

5

THE ELEPHANT IN THE ROOM – MENTAL HEALTH ILLNESS IN CHILDREN AND YOUNG PEOPLE

Can health play specialists make a difference?

Irene O'Donnell – NHS Hospital Trust lead for therapeutic play, recreation and youth services

The number of children and young people (CYP) requiring urgent help and support for their mental health is at crisis point – the exact same point as them. According to the Mental Health Foundation, mental health difficulties in CYP usually develop early with 50 percent established by the age of 14 and 75 percent by young adulthood (MHF, 2022).

It was highlighted by the mental health survey (2017) that one in every nine CYP between the ages of 5 and 15 years old had a diagnosable mental disorder (NHS Digital, 2018). From a follow-up NHS survey undertaken in 2021, the extent of children with mental disorders had increased to one in six (NHS Digital, 2021). Some groups of CYP are more at risk of developing mental health problems such as children in social care, those with serious physical health problems or chronic illness, children with disabilities or learning difficulties, neurodevelopmental conditions such as autism and those living in poverty (Faulconbridge et al., 2019).

The growing trajectory of mental health illness in CYP over the past decade is a worrying situation made even more concerning as the services to support the needs of these CYP have not grown at the same rate as their mental illness. This has left many general paediatric units around the UK having increasing numbers of admissions of CYP in mental health crisis. Staff often feel overwhelmed and out of their depth to support these young people and can lack knowledge and confidence to enable them to provide the appropriate support and environment (Duggan, 2022).

It is easy to identify a pattern as to why so many CYP are now presenting to emergency departments to seek the help that they are unable to access via primary health services such as GP services or Child Adolescent Mental Health Services (CAMHS). Many parents and carers state that they are left with little choice other than to turn to their local emergency department when they are dealing with their

DOI: 10.4324/9781003255444-7

child in crisis. When a child or young person is spiralling into deeper illness and distress families are often desperate for someone to help them. The mental health charity Young Minds (2022) shares that support and treatment is not readily available or easy to access when it is most needed, leaving many to manage alone.

They also highlight much longer-term consequences to CYP not being able to access mental health support at the point of need. If early intervention and help is not received then there is a risk of young people's mental health problems deepening, requiring more acute and costly interventions and having a serious impact on their lives (Duggan, 2022). According to Duggan CYP mental health services have been historically underfunded. Although work has started to make improvements to services, and there has been an increase in training of the workforce, it will take considerable time to start to see the impact and benefits of this.

As concerning as the data might be, it would be balanced by a reassurance that timely support at the point of need would be available to all who needed it. Sadly, this is far from the reality facing CYP and their families in the UK today.

So, what are the reasons for this? For example, if you break your leg you can go to your local emergency department and present for the urgent care you require. Would the medical and nursing team tell you they have no one available to see you and that you will be triaged in the next few years? Of course not – but this highlights the stark contrast between services for physical and mental health illness and the inequality and lack of parity of care that coexists in the funding of health services (Kings Fund, 2022).

It is also a strange but familiar idea that physical and mental health are two separate entities, that you can somehow treat one or the other in a silo. Many CYP will struggle with physical symptoms caused by their mental health illness such as headaches, pain and sleep problems with no organic cause (Faulconbridge et al., 2019).

Adolescence and mental health

Adolescence can be a time of turmoil when young people enter puberty, which can be a catalyst for mental ill health. Hormone changes can ignite mood swings, rage and overwhelm CYPs with difficulty regulating emotions. Along with huge changes physically and emotionally in how young people are living, the rise of social media use is exposing many young people to risks of poor mental health and well-being (Mayo Clinic, 2022). The most common mental health problems that CYP experience are anxiety disorders including obsessive-compulsive disorder (OCD), depression, self-harm and eating disorders (Duggan, 2022).

Adolescence can be an increased time of vulnerability for those with neurodevelopmental conditions such as autism spectrum disorder (ASD) or Attention Deficit Hyperactivity Disorder (ADHD), who are already at an increased risk of developing mental health problems (Faulconbridge et al., 2019). The charity Autistica states seven out of ten autistic people will experience a mental health illness or difficulty (Mental Health Foundation, 2022). ADHD affects mood, behaviour and executive function skills which can lead to feelings of being overwhelmed especially at exam time or other stresses and transitions (Young Minds, 2022).

Trauma can impact on our mental health and emotional well-being. Adverse childhood experiences (ACEs), such as abuse, neglect and household dysfunction, are considered to increase the likelihood of the rate of mental health problems later in life (Faulconbridge et al., 2019). One in three adults who have experienced an ACE will develop a mental health illness (Manchester University NHS Foundation Trust, 2022).

The role of the health play specialist

Health play specialists (HPSs) are highly skilled professionals who manage complex situations with children/young people and their families on a frequent basis (HPSET, 2022a). A skilled practitioner who can support a CYP with their emotional intelligence enables them to explore experiences through play and gain a better understanding of their feelings and those of others (O'Donnell, 2012).

Working with CYP can be very rewarding and bring a great sense of purpose in helping others to overcome challenges with their health. But it can also be challenging on occasions, particularly when presented with a CYP who is struggling with mental ill health. It's easy to feel out of your depth, wonder what to say and how to support a young person to feel comfortable sharing their feelings and worries about their mental health (Young Minds, 2022).

HPSs approach from an advantageous position of being non-clinical and can feel like a safe trusting person to engage with. Playful activity for joy, boredom or distraction can be hugely beneficial and a therapeutic tool (Brown, 2016). It can enable CYP to navigate their mental health illness and recover their well-being enhancing emotional intelligence and agility. Delivering therapeutic play and activity in healthcare can be utilised for all CYP regardless of their diagnosis. Whether you work as a HPS or a youth support coordinator (YSC) it takes kindness, empathy and patience to work with CYP with mental health illness – the same skills needed for being a HPS working with all CYP with physical health illness.

So why do CYP who have a mental health illness rather than a physical health illness feel more daunting – the elephant in the room? Some possible reasons may be the fear of mental ill health, the stigma (sometimes unconscious bias) that is still attached to mental ill health and the lack of confidence in knowing what to say or do. It can feel frustrating to offer help to CYP who are not willing (or ready) to accept it. It can look like the CYP is well and even appear that they have everything they need – caring parents, a loving home and a comfortable life. They may have no physical health conditions that many young people in the other beds around the ward are struggling with daily and would do whatever it takes to stop. Some may still have a view that mental ill health is a choice and that the CYP could prevent ending up in crisis, self-harming, or suicide attempts and are a drain on the already strained overworked and busy NHS resources. These are real feelings and thoughts that exist within society and healthcare. To enable positive change, we must challenge these ideas by understating more about mental health illness and work in partnership with CYP and their families.

It can be helpful to attend debriefs and multidisciplinary team meetings which brings the chance for the HPS to share experience and work in collaboration to plan care for CYP and their families (Faulconbridge et al., 2019). Taking opportunities to write up a reflection of supporting CYP with their mental health can enable reflective practice learning and form part of the evidence needed for re-registration for HPSs (HPSET, 2022b). Requesting clinical supervision if available enables support for HPSs and practitioners own mental health and resilience, which is crucial to enabling the work needed to deliver this care on a regular ongoing basis.

For many CYP talking to a formal mental health professional can feel overwhelming, stigmatising or frightening at first, especially if they are in crisis. Therapeutic activity can be a vessel for engaging with CYP and helping them process in a safe contained way. Many young people will have experienced trauma so the adults in their lives are critical in helping them cope when they're struggling (Young Minds, 2022) (Figure 5.1).

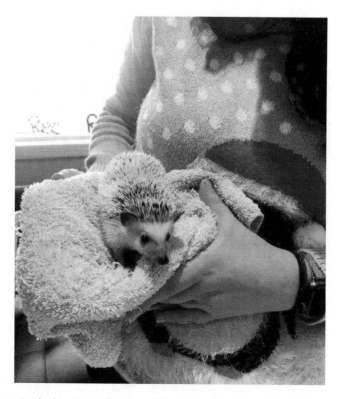

FIGURE 5.1 Hedgehog Betty from a wild science visit.

Conclusion: the way forward

There is no doubt progress is being made and attitudes to mental ill health have improved over the past few years, but there is still some way to go. Having a better understanding of your own mental health will equip you to be better placed at supporting other peoples' challenging issues (NHS, 2022). That will help in supporting the CYP the same as you would when approaching a CYP diagnosed with a physical health condition. Increasing knowledge from training initiatives will also help, such as *We Can Talk* (Healthy Teen Minds, 2022), which is a co-designed and delivered training for healthcare staff to help improve the experience of CYP who attend hospital due to their mental health. Feedback from staff has been positive, e.g. an increased confidence in staff supporting CYP in mental health crisis and having conversations about mental health. Knowledge is power.

Underneath the mental illness is a CYP, a human being that is probably very frightened and in physical and emotional pain and distress. Play specialists have multiple transferable skills to support CYP with mental ill health. HPSs are often in a privileged position of building rapport and trust which enables a therapeutic relationship. Play is healing on so many levels and in its simplest form is joyful, relaxing and cathartic (Brown, 2010) (Figure 5.2).

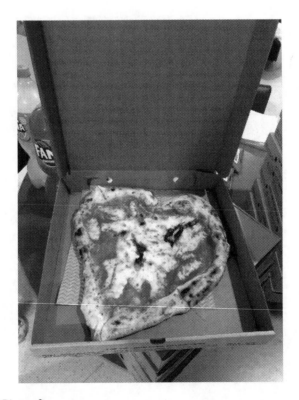

FIGURE 5.2 Pizza afternoon.

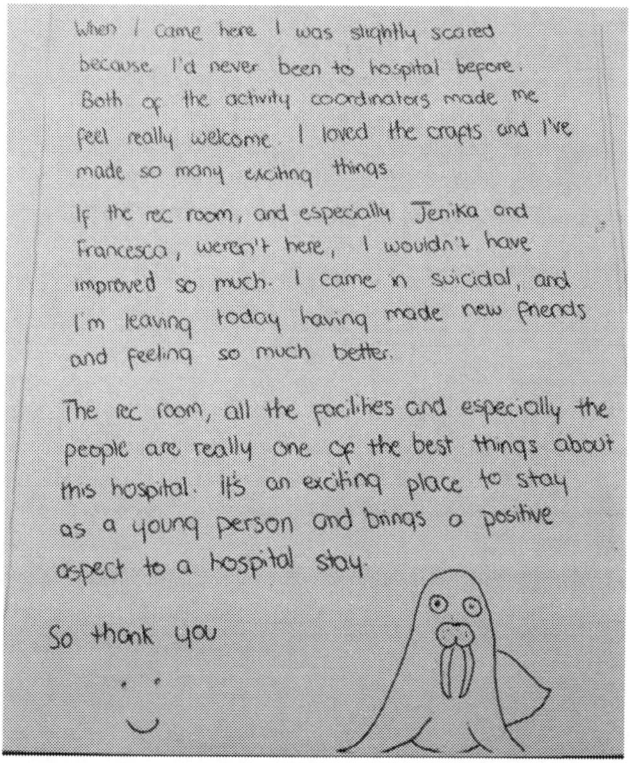

When I came here I was slightly scared because I'd never been to hospital before. Both of the activity coordinators made me feel really welcome. I loved the crafts and I've made so many exciting things.

If the rec room, and especially Jenika and Francesca, weren't here, I wouldn't have improved so much. I came in suicidal, and I'm leaving today having made new friends and feeling so much better.

The rec room, all the facilities and especially the people are really one of the best things about this hospital. It's an exciting place to stay as a young person and brings a positive aspect to a hospital stay.

So thank you

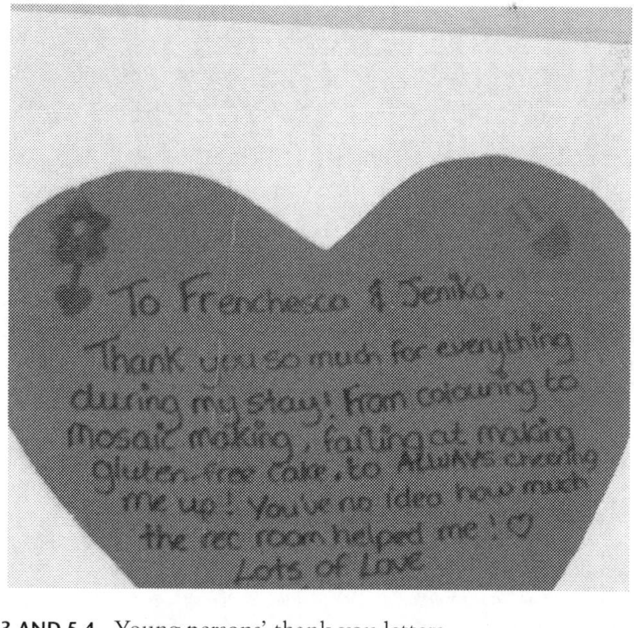

To Frenchesca & Jenika,

Thank you so much for everything during my stay! From colouring to mosaic making, failing at making gluten-free cake, to Always cheering me up! You've no idea how much the rec room helped me! ♡

Lots of Love

FIGURES 5.3 AND 5.4 Young persons' thank you letters.

Early intervention is key to reducing the chances of mental ill health escalating, so the implementation of training, funding and resources from the UK government are welcome and timely to avoid any further escalation of a mental health crisis in our youth. Every CYP should have the opportunity to make informed decisions about their own mental health care and treatment, working alongside family and professionals to decide what is best for them (Anna Freud NCCF, 2022). Prompt access to appropriate support enables CYP experiencing difficulties to maximise their prospects for a healthy and happy life (NHS Digital, 2021).

Together we can make a positive difference to a child or young person in distress – whatever the cause of the distress is. For many years it has been acknowledged that safeguarding is everyone's business and not just for those specialists working in the child protection arena. Adopting a similar approach and attitude to CYPs mental health – it is everybody's business – could be the start of further breaking down stigma and fear and offering support at the point of need.

HPSs are often the right people, in the right place, at the right time to support CYP who are unwell with their mental health. Highly skilled and trained in therapeutic play, we can make a positive difference to the experience of all CYP in healthcare, regardless of the illness or condition. Health play specialists can lead the way in supporting CYP through therapeutic play and skills to build resilience and manage emotions. Play is seriously good for your health and the recipients agree (see Figures 5.3 and 5.4). Let's let the elephant out of the room.

References

Anna Freud NCCF (2022) *Shared Decision Making Poster.* Anna Freud National Centre for Children and Families. [Online] Available from: <https://www.annafreud.org/media/10347/sdm-poster-final-3.pdf> [Accessed 16 June 2022]

Brown, F. (2016) The Healing Power of Play: therapeutic work with chronically neglected and abused children. In: Navidi, U. ed. (2016) *The Role of Play in Children's Health and Development.* Basel: MDPI

Brown, S. (2010) *Play: How It Shapes the Brain Opens the Imagination and Invigorates the Soul.* Harmondsworth: Penguin

Duggan, S. (2022) *Tackling the Increase in Demand for Mental Health Support in Children and Young People.* NHS Confederation. [Online] Available from: <https://www.nhsconfed.org/articles/tackling-increase-demand-mental-health-support-children-and-young-people> [Accessed 16 June 2022]

Faulconbridge, J., Hunt, K. & Laffan, A. eds. (2019) *Improving the Psychological Wellbeing of Children and Young People.* London: Jessica Kingsley Publishers

Healthy Teen Minds (2022) *We Can Talk.* [Online] Available from: <https://wecantalk.online/> [Accessed 16 June 2022]

HPSET (2022a) *Training and Entry.* [Online] Available from: <https://hpset.org.uk/training-entry/> [Accessed 15 May 2022]

HPSET (2022b) *Annual Re-Registration Guide.* [Online] Available from: https://hpset.org.uk/registration/ [Accessed 16 June 2022]

Kings Fund (2022) *Has the Government Put Mental Health on an Equal Footing with Physical Health?* [Online] Available from: <https://www.kingsfund.org.uk/projects/verdict/has-government-put-mental-health-equal-footing-physical-health> [Accessed 26 June 2022]

Manchester University NHS Foundation Trust (2022) *Adverse Childhood Experiences (ACEs) and Attachment.* [Online] Available from: <https://mft.nhs.uk/rmch/services/camhs/young-people/adverse-childhood-experiences-aces-and-attachment/> [Accessed 26 June 2022]

Mayo Clinic (2022) *Teens and Social Media Use: What's the Impact?* [Online] Available from: <https://www.mayoclinic.org/healthy-lifestyle/tween-and-teen-health/in-depth/teens-and-social-media-use/art-20474437#> [Accessed 16 June 2022]

Mental Health Foundation (MHF) (2022) *Autism and Mental Health.* [Online] Available from: <https://www.mentalhealth.org.uk/a-to-z/a/autism-and-mental-health> [Accessed 26 June 2022]

NHS (2022) *Every Mind Matters.* [Online] Available from: <https://www.nhs.uk/every-mind-matters/supporting-others/helping-others/> [Accessed 26 June 2022]

NHS Digital (2018) *Mental Health of Children and Young People in England 2017.* [Online] Available from: <https://www.gov.uk/government/statistics/mental-health-of-children-and-young-people-in-england-2017-pas> [Accessed 15 June 2022]

NHS Digital (2021) *Mental Health of Children and Young People in England 2021 – Wave 2 Follow up to the 2017 Survey.* [Online] Available from: <https://digital.nhs.uk/data-and-information/publications/statistical/mental-health-of-children-and-young-people-in-england/2021-follow-up-to-the-2017-survey> [Accessed 15 June 2022]

O'Donnell, I. (2012) Profile of new committee member. *The Journal of the National Association of Hospital Play Staff,* Issue 50, Spring 2012, pp. 9–10

Young Minds (2022) *Fighting for Young People's Mental Health.* [Online] Available from: <https://www.youngminds.org.uk/> [Accessed 16 June 2022]

6

THE HOSPITAL PLAYROOM

A key part of children and young people's care and recovery

David Stonehouse – Senior Lecturer

Introduction

The hospital playroom has been an important part of children's wards since the early 1960s. This chapter will first discuss the background and importance of play for children and young people in hospital and the role that the playroom provides. The chapter then moves on to examine a piece of research undertaken by the author, examining the experience of participants studying on pre-registration children's nursing degree courses regarding the use of playrooms on children's wards. Results will be presented and discussed. Conclusions and recommendations will be made, before highlighting the implications for children's wards and children's nurses worldwide.

Background

"Play is an essential part of every child's life" (Play England, 2020), with Tondatti and Correa (2012) stating it is the most important activity. Play is characterised by fun, challenge, flexibility, uncertainty and non-productivity (United Nations International Children's Emergency Fund, 2014). When children and young people become ill and require hospital admission, play becomes important as a link to home and as a way for the child to take control of often a difficult and potentially distressing situation (Hubbuck, 2009). Play also delivers many benefits for children in hospital; from speeding up recovery and rehabilitation and reducing the need for some medical interventions needing to be performed under general anaesthesia (Jun-Tai, 2004, 2008) to self-expression, enabling children to express their feelings and emotions (Brown & Patte, 2013).

DOI: 10.4324/9781003255444-8

The importance of the hospital playroom within the United Kingdom was first officially highlighted within the Platt Report (Ministry of Health, 1959). This report recognised that all children's wards needed a playroom, which was visible to the children from their hospital beds. Play Wales (2015) echoed this point 56 years later stating that having a playroom sends a strong message that children have permission to play whilst in hospital.

Hubbuck (2009, p. 142) states the case more strongly suggesting the playroom is "a haven for sick children", with Weinberger et al. (2017) calling the playroom a refuge. Crenshaw and Kelly (2018) also state that the purpose of the playroom is to give children and families moments of non-demanding, untethered and spontaneous joy.

Though Weinberger et al.'s (2017) research into hospital playroom design in America focused on the internal environment, they did identify that the nature element was also very important. Windows providing lots of natural light with views of trees and grass benefit children and adults alike. Play Wales (2015) also stresses the importance of children having access to outdoor play spaces which can provide a place of solace from the ward environment. Therefore, a playroom with access to the outside environment is important. Play Wales (2015) repeats the recommendations made by Bird (2007, p. 6) who states that contact with nature can be "an effective component of coping with anxiety and stress, particularly for patients undergoing operations".

Research

Longitudinal focus groups were used to gain data from participants recruited from two UK universities who were undertaking a pre-registration children's nursing degree. Longitudinal focus groups were chosen over one-off focus groups, to discover if opinions changed regarding play as participants progressed through both the educational setting and clinical practice components of their course.

Results

In discussing the two questions, "How has the playroom been used?" and "Who has used it and for what?" 55% of participants stated that the playroom was often used for something other than play. Thirty-five per cent said medical assessments as well as blood samples were taken by the doctor in the playroom. Twenty per cent of participants stated that in their opinion the playroom was not big enough, with a further 10% stating that the playroom was often shared with another area.

One participant stated:

> I think my perception before of a children's ward was where kids went into the playroom and played or whatever, you do not see that at all.

They went on to say that perhaps it was the fault of the staff who do not encourage parents to take their children into the playroom.

> We do not encourage parents necessarily to go and take their kids to the playroom, like every kid needs to be in bed on the ward do they, they can go off… because that is what they would do at home they would go off and play and do their own thing and why can't they, they do not really do that the same.

A further participant discussed the fact that the playroom was only open Monday to Friday 09:00 to 17:00 and shut during mealtimes. Outside of those hours it was locked, with no access in the evening, overnight or at weekends. Despite having an outside play area with equipment, this was never seen to be used even in warm weather. However, in contrast one participant stated that the outdoor play area on their placement was used, with staff encouraging children to go outside in the fresh air and even ride bikes.

Also on a positive note, one participant stated:

> The playroom was open all the time. It was open 24/7 even at night the doors were open just in case anyone came in late at night or someone was really distressed they would go in the playroom. It is quite well used for the long term patients I found, because obviously the parents by then are quite comfortable to just go in and use whatever they want and they had a sensory area so any children with sensory impairments could go and sit in that area, and the play therapist would just encourage people to go in or just be like a support in the playroom, but I found that most of the time the parents would go in there with their children.

A surprising finding was that just over half of participants had witnessed the hospital playroom being used for other things than play. One participant stated on their surgical placement, the playroom was used to perform the pre-operative checks the patients had prior to undergoing their operations. A second participant said that on a similar ward the surgeons would speak to the parents in the playroom, whilst a third participant said the playroom was used as a waiting room for parents waiting for their children to return from surgery.

Discussion

The importance of hospital playrooms within the UK was identified 60 years ago in the Platt Report (Ministry of Health, 1959, p. 10):

> All children's wards need a playroom, preferably visible to the children in bed. Noise can be cut off by glass screens, but the sick child derives a stimulus to get better from seeing others play.

Fifty years later Hubbuck (2009, p. 142) describes the playroom as "a haven for sick children". She suggests they provide a means for reducing boredom and thereby decreasing stress and anxiety. They allow children to make positive choices with what they can do with their time, giving back to them a sense of control. They also give the child the chance to socialise and communicate with their peers sharing their experiences (Hubbuck, 2009).

In examining playrooms in Ireland, Crenshaw and Kelly (2018) identified that playrooms were designed according to the ward's speciality, with toys selected appropriately. They stated that the purpose of each playroom was "to give children and their families a moment of spontaneous, non-demanding, and untethered joy" (Crenshaw & Kelly, 2018, p. 61). Children there had free choice in what they choose to play with, and how they played.

Within the focus groups, participants highlighted that the playroom was not always the haven which Hubbuck (2009) states it should be. Just over half of the participants stated that the playroom was often used for something other than play with a third of participants reporting that medical assessments were performed by doctors in the playroom and one participant stated they had witnessed blood being taken from a child there. This goes directly against what Weinberger et al. (2017, p. 72) propose, that "playrooms serve as a refuge for children, and while the absence of medical tests and procedures in playrooms sets the stage, playrooms can be more than a shelter from medical intervention".

If this is the case, then it demonstrates a lack of awareness of the hospital staff in the importance of play for children in hospital and the role that the playroom can provide in this.

Other participants also stated that the playroom was used as a storeroom and as a waiting room. This clearly identifies that hospital playrooms are not always being used in the way they have been planned and designed to be used (Hubbuck, 2009; Weinberger et al., 2017). Perhaps more significantly, playrooms are not being valued by healthcare professionals for the contribution to children's happiness that they bring. This could be down to pressure of space within a children's ward, the convenience of the member of staff performing the intervention or lack of awareness and training in the importance of play for children in hospital.

On a positive note, one participant did state that the playroom they saw on placement was open access and children and their families could use it at any time, day or night. However, this was not the experience of everyone with some playrooms being locked when the Health Play Specialist was not on duty.

Play Wales (2015) clearly asserted that having a hospital playroom sends a strong message that children have permission to play whilst in hospital. However, the implication of the playroom being used inappropriately for medical investigations, as a waiting room or as a storeroom is that it makes it clear that play is not important within that area. The correct use of playrooms for the purposes of providing a haven (Hubbuck, 2009) and a refuge (Weinberger et al., 2017) in which children can play needs to be taken back from the improper uses that they are being used for. It would seem that nurses need to advocate for this haven and refuge to be utilised for the purpose it has been designed and protect it from misuse.

Conclusions/recommendations

The author has researched the use of playrooms within clinical healthcare areas within the UK. It is clear there is inconsistency in the way playrooms are used. Participants identified that some playrooms were no longer the refuge they were designed to be. Participants also reported that children were not utilising the playroom as much as they thought they would. Nurses acting as the advocates for their patients need, in collaboration with Health Play Specialists and other staff, to take back the playroom for children's play. Playrooms should not be used to conduct interviews and assessments of patients and their family members. Nor should they be used to perform invasive clinical procedures which by their nature are often distressing and painful to children. Neither should the playroom be used as a meeting room for clinical staff or as a storeroom. Children should have open access to the playroom whenever they need to. There would also appear to be a need to raise awareness with hospital staff regarding the importance of play for children in hospital.

Implications for children's wards worldwide

This chapter has focused on playrooms within children's wards in the UK. However, the implications can be significant for all staff caring for children within a hospital environment anywhere in the world. There needs to be an examination of the play facilities on children's wards to make sure they are not being abused and children are receiving the play opportunities they deserve and need.

References

Bird, W. (2007) *Natural thinking: investigating the links between the natural environment, biodiversity and mental health.* [Online]. Royal Society for the Protection of Birds. Available from: http://ww2.rspb.org.uk [Accessed 18 October 2021].

Brown, F. & Patte, M. (2013) *Rethinking children's play.* London: Bloomsbury.

Crenshaw, D.A. & Kelly, J.E. (2018) Play therapy in assisting children with medical challenges. In: Rubin, L. C. (Ed.), *Handbook of medical play therapy and child life.* London: Routledge, pp. 57–68.

Hubbuck, C. (2009) *Play for sick children: play specialists in hospital and beyond.* London: Jessica Kingsley Publishers.

Jun-Tai, N. (2004) *Factsheet No. 6 play in hospital.* [Online]. Children's Play Information Service. Available from: http://docplayer.net/20755599-No-6-play-in-hospital.html [Accessed 18 October 2021].

Jun-Tai, N. (2008) Play in hospital. *Paediatrics and Child Health*, 18 (5), pp. 233–237. https://doi.org/10.1016/j.paed.2008.02.002.

Ministry of Health (1959) *The welfare of children in hospital*. London: Her Majesty's Stationary Office.

Play England (2020) *Charter for play*. [Online]. Play England. Available from: http://www.playengland.org.uk [Accessed 18 October 2021].

Play Wales (2015) *Hospital play*. [Online]. Play Wales. Available from: http://www.play-wales.org.uk [Accessed 18 October 2021].

Tondatti, P. C. & Correa, I. (2012) Use of music and play in pediatric nursing care in the hospital context. *Investigación Educación Enfermería*, 30 (3), pp. 362–370. http://ref.scielo.org/w5jcgg

UNICEF (2014) *General comments of the committee on the rights of the child: a compendium for child rights advocates, scholars and policy makers*. [Online]. United Nations International Children's Emergency Fund. Available from: https://www.unicef.org [Accessed 18 October 2021].

Weinberger, N., Butler, A., McGee, B., Schumacher, P. & Brown, R. (2017) Child life specialists' evaluation of hospital playroom design: a mixed method inquiry. *Journal of Interior Design*, 42 (2), pp. 71–91. https://doi.org/10.1111/joid.12097.

PART II

Personal reflections on the role of the hospital play specialist

7

MY JOURNEY

*Lisa Beaumont – Therapeutic and
Specialised Play Manager*

So where did my journey begin, how did I become a Therapeutic and Specialist
Service manager at Leeds Children's Hospital with numerous awards and a medal
from the queen!

I have always loved being around children, from the age of 12 years old, I use
to knock on neighbours' doors and ask if I could take their babies for a walk …
which they would let me! Of course, I always returned them after a trip around
the local park. Leaving school, I could not decide between childcare or catering,
as my dad said to me, "people will always need someone to look after their children and people will always want to eat". I chose to work with children!

I saw a job advertised in the local paper, advertising for a Nursery Nurse in
Leeds, at St James Hospital. This sparked my interest and reminded me of the
many times I had spent, as a child in hospital, where I would spend long periods
of time just waiting for my parents to come and visit me, unable to get off my
bed, with long periods of boredom. So, I decided to apply for the job. I was inter-
viewed by the ward sister in a large white hat, a blue starched uniform with a big
shiny buckle belt and I somehow convinced her to give me the job.

Back then, play was not high on the ward manager's agenda; in fact, it was not
high on anyone's agenda within the hospital. I became part of a wonderful ward
team that worked closely together every day. I was the only play staff/nursery
nurse at that time on the medical ward, with one other nursery nurse working
in oncology funded by a charity, whereas I was funded by the National Health
Service (NHS).

It was not easy working on a very busy medical ward with a Sister, who ran
a very tight ship, and staff having little knowledge then around the importance
of play. I started my role on the ward with a packet of felt tip pens that the ward
clerk managed to order for me. Then over the next few years I managed to move
from my own shelf to a cupboard, followed by a small play space, then a small

DOI: 10.4324/9781003255444-10

playroom, to a larger playroom where I ran daily activities, from water play to baking. I found a love for working with children with Cystic Fibrosis and always welcomed an opportunity to try and tempt their appetites with baking. From pizzas to pancakes, we did it all, including setting off the fire alarm one morning while having a pancake breakfast party! I remember shrinking in my shoes as the Matron came marching onto the ward 'to tell me off'!

There were many photographs displayed on the walls of the children/young people who had visited our ward regularly, and of those we had lost. They became a wall of memories over the years, as we moved wards, departments, and hospitals (see Figure 7.1).

I really felt for the children with a Cystic Fibrosis diagnosis; often they would spend many months in hospital away from their family and friends. I worked

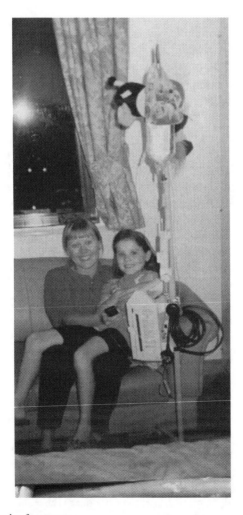

FIGURE 7.1   Not to be forgotten.

hard to be creative in offering a variety of activities. When children could not socialise or mix, I bought walkie talkies to help keep that link with others and when parents could not visit. I would prioritise those children that needed me most, which was not easy on such a busy ward and with so many children. I did my best to see each child and young person where I could and bring some fun to their day, while ensuring where possible to continue to raise the profile of my specialised role to the medical staff that I worked with; convincing the doctors to use me during discussions or procedures; and to shout for me so I could work alongside them to prepare or distract children where possible. This is something some of us still struggle with today!

I felt I could be seen as being a nuisance by some of the junior doctors – what was my singing and bubble-blowing going to achieve? I saw it all the time with consultants, often too busy or maybe less interested to acknowledge my thoughts or role. However, after working hard with all the professionals over many years, I slowly became recognised, and colleagues began to believe in what I could do and deliver. I still had to explain I could not perform magic or fix the impossible and being called to support in a timely manner was key to my success!

Many of the team from my early days, such as the junior staff, have now moved to senior staff and even management and can still recall the difference we made and the need to have a good play service in place, as it made such a difference to the children's and young person's journey/hospital admission. Things have now changed and moved on to some extent. However, in general terms Play in Hospital, and its value, still continues to be an ongoing fight. In some areas and hospitals, it is not seen as a priority and there is still more work to be done.

In 1999, along with the support of the ward manager and one of the band six sisters, we set up a charity to help grant children wishes for children with Cystic Fibrosis as we felt this was a little bit of a forgotten illness and in those days a very sad one. We achieved this and it became a real success, we were able to send a couple of children to America, some went on shopping trips and some on theatre visits. However, something that I will remember forever, is that I had one little girl who dreamed of being a bridesmaid, so she became just that for my own wedding. Unfortunately, this little girl passed away a few years later but it still gives me great pleasure to think of making her dream come true on my wedding day.

I have worked with so many inspirational children, and sadly seen many lose their fight. End of life support was an aspect of my role, and this would often happen on the ward. I would sit with many of them in their final days trying to hold back my emotions, I would read to them, and we would talk about our favourite subjects over the years. This part of my role has always been hard to explain, and something I will always struggle to get my head around, nothing can prepare you for the loss of a child.

In 1994, my brother was killed in a Road Traffic Accident by a drunk driver. The loss and emotional grief, which I had never felt before, was something I thought I would never be able to get over, and I began to worry that I would not be able to continue in this line of work. However, thankfully I did and in 1995 the ward manager agreed that I could do the Hospital Play Specialist course. I had to pay the course fees myself as there was no funding then, and I had to travel to Bolton College on my day off. The ward manager was supportive and agreed that I could work Sundays so I could go to Bolton each Tuesday on my day off to complete my studies.

Once I had completed the Hospital Play Specialist course, the Trust was asked to consider developing a Children's Liver Transplant service, one of only three in the country. We worked hard as a team to develop and start to deliver a super-regional service for Children's Liver Transplants. I recall this work as some of the finest work I have ever been involved in, with surgeons, consultants, and psychologists all really valuing the role of the Health Play Specialist. One surgeon would come to me every morning and asked me how his patients were, always keen to know how they had engaged in the daily activities, while responding to treatment or recovering from surgery.

Preparing children and young people became one of the many focal points in my daily work, alongside distraction for endless requests for blood tests. I also developed role play materials and a variety of preparation materials, one of which is transplant teddies which are still being used today. The children love to build a bear with us, giving them a green coloured small liver, which is to indicate that the liver is not 'too well' like theirs, then replacing this green liver with a nice new pink one, just like they receive during their transplant. I started this idea when asked to prepare a young child who would have really struggled to understand what was to come, I remember how his mum explained that it had been taken to nursery and how the child had explained that his teddy like him, was getting a new liver (see Figure 7.2).

The next few years saw us to continue to develop a range of preparation and distraction clinics for our transplant children. I continued to engage the children in positive activities after organ transplant and I became the team manager for 'Leeds Little Livers' a group of children who had liver transplants, we helped to support and encourage children to take part in the British Transplant Games, this is an event where Transplanted Children come together each year from across the many transplant centres and we celebrate the gift of life while giving thanks to their Donor families. I'm proud to say the team is now called Leeds Children Transplant team and has children who have had liver, kidney, and bone marrow transplants. We have come such a long way.

We have also taken part in activity camps at TACKERS in Switzerland, an international camp for transplant children where they would spend an amazing week up a mountain. Seeing these children and young people after long periods of time in hospital was just so rewarding. The children have some really amazing experiences during this time such as skiing, dog sledging, or making new friends, which is all run by a lady called Liz who had a transplant as an adult herself. This camp was supported by a variety of transplant nurses and doctors from the transplant units across the country.

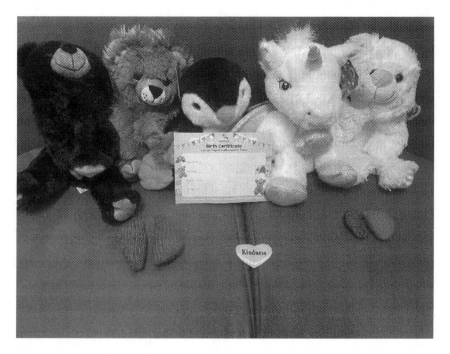

FIGURE 7.2 Transplant teddies.

Over the next few years, we also centralised as a children's service over at the Leeds General Infirmary where we then said goodbye to the many years at St James Hospital. Soon the Agenda for Change was introduced within the NHS, which was an unsettling time for the play service, and we all had to reapply for our own jobs. There were many changes and developments happening I was able to take on one of the more senior play specialist roles, as medical lead part time.

I have worked with a great team of Health Play Specialists and Play Leaders, and a few years ago I was very excited to see the management team had recognised that there was a need for a play service lead. I was over the moon to be the successful candidate for this role with the title of: Therapeutic and Specialised Play Service Manager, I would never have thought all those years ago I would have the privilege to hold such a role.

I would never have thought many years ago that I would be where I am today, but I know that it is a job that challenges me every day, I always think of the child at the centre of every meeting or report I may be asked to review or write. The children in the hospital and the service we provide will continue to develop and grow, while supporting the child/young person's hospital journey.

Over the years I have received a number of awards and nominations; each and every one makes me proud and for those that know me, very emotional.

I see each one as an opportunity to raise our profile and the role within play. However, more than anything I have accepted these awards over the years in memory of the many children that have lost their fight against a whole range of childhood diseases and illness, along with their families they are the true heroes and always will be and will always be remembered. I have kept some lovely things from families over the years, often cards, photos, or a few lines on a note, I will treasure them always.

I just love what I do, I always have, and I always will. Not many people get to spend their whole life doing what they love and for that I am always grateful.

8

THE 'MAGIC OF PLAY'

Exploring the importance of play and distraction during medical procedures

Katie Lane – Health Play Specialist

Play and distraction provided by a qualified play specialist (HPS) has a place during medical procedures (Walker, 2006; Hubbuck, 2009; Tonkin, 2014). Sometimes it is the main focus for the HPS's involvement in a patient's care. At other times, HPSs are ready and waiting for the right moment to engage or distract.

Evidence which explores and promotes the importance of play during medical procedures is limited (Tonkin, 2014; Perasso et al., 2021). In some cases, it can be hard to know how a child would have responded to an invasive, painful procedure without the additional input of the HPS. Even when the HPS is present and providing play interventions, not all children successfully engage or complete procedures because some just do not – or cannot due to their extreme anxiety or distress. What HPSs do is offer a safe and appropriate environment in which children can undergo procedures with the positive presence of the HPS to advocate for them and support them before, during and after these stressful situations.

In this chapter, I share a memory of a procedure and the support I provided to a child who was an inpatient in a children's hospital setting. I explore how my professional input impacted the experience of that procedure for the child, parent and medical professionals present. I also give a narrative to the 'working method' used by HPSs and highlight the challenges they face when providing play support to children and young people undergoing invasive medical procedures. In presenting this case study I have changed the names of those involved. I tell the story in separate parts and discuss the child's experience, and the HPS's approach between each part.

DOI: 10.4324/9781003255444-11

I meet Ron and his mother and introduce myself and my role as a HPS on the ward. His nurse says that when members of staff enter his cubicle, he won't make eye contact, or vocalise in any way, and withdraws from what he was doing. After some positive interactions with me, including engaging in play, Ron began to engage more and became more confident in vocalising how he was feeling and what he wanted to do.

After sharing these positive play experiences with Ron and his mum, I could see Ron was noticing the difference between my role and that of the doctors and nurses.

The 'magic of play'. That is what some people call it; and certainly a couple of engrossing activities which include lots of laughter and silliness can allow a child to feel comfortable around the HPS. Part of the skill is to assess a child, get down to their level and quickly establish both what they need and what they like, and – in doing so – to start creating a relationship of trust. It may look like 'magic', but it is not as simple as that. These powerful play interactions allow the HPS to access a child's world – to see their personality and their way of thinking. Through play, the HPS starts to learn more about a child, how they like to explore, what they like and dislike.

Sometimes play with the HPS may be loud, fast and physical – other times quiet and focused on a task. Soon enough, most children begin to behave more openly, showing enthusiasm – and showing when they are frightened or anxious or angry. Ron started to greet me by my name. He would jump up and down on his bed when he saw me getting prepared outside his cubical. As our relationship of trust developed, it was terrific to see him so happy to see someone in a uniform enter his room. This was not the case for other medical professionals.

When admitted to hospital, Ron was four years old. He has epilepsy and was admitted due to an increase in seizure activity. His seizures varied in type and length, from 5 to 10 seconds to a couple of minutes. When we first met, Ron had already undergone several invasive and distressing medical interventions without a HPS present.

A couple of intense seizures had led to Ron falling and hurting himself. He had started to feel scared about getting down from his bed and was worried about falling again. Ron's medical team had decided that due to the increased intensity of his seizures Ron needed central intravenous (IV) access. Previous attempts to cannulate Ron had proved tricky due to his small veins, and led to him experiencing multiple attempts to cannulate. Consequently, Ron now became very upset and cross when medical professionals approached him. He resisted all invasive and non-invasive procedures and interventions, including having observations done (oxygen saturations, blood pressure and temperature). Ron's mum was struggling to cope with seeing Ron go through these distressing procedures and decided not to be present.

As I enter Ron is lying across his mum's lap. Dr Trelawny is attempting to insert a cannula into his right foot.

Ron is in and out of focal seizures and crying. He is trying to wiggle out of mum's comfort hold. Mum is leaning off the bed trying to comfort Ron and hold him still with no additional support.

I politely ask "What is going on in here?"

Dr Trelawny replies "Failing to get access".

I ask, 'How many attempts have there been?' and discover she is about to try Ron's right foot for the second time, having previously attempting to access a vein in his hand. No local anaesthetic has been applied to either area, presumably due to the urgency of him needing IV access.

In a bouncy but serious voice I suggest Ron and mum need a break and together we need to rethink the plan.

Dr Trelawny puts the cannula back in the tray, saying she will contact the consultant to decide on the next steps, she leaves the cubicle.

I check-in with Ron and mum and help get them comfy on his bed. They have a cuddle and Ron starts to calm down, but he does not look over at me or communicate with me at all.

HPSs undergo two years of training – a combination of in-depth theoretical learning about child development and the effects of hospitalisation on children, and practical placements. These involve a considerable amount of observation and continuous reflective practice. This continues into professional practice, where their theoretical knowledge is deepened by frequent encounters with children and families in intense, high-stress situations, including the kind of procedure experienced by Ron.

The HPS's knowledge and skills inform the way they behave and respond to the needs of children. There are numerous things happening in these encounters that only become apparent when reflecting on the experience. The HPS role relies on both acquired knowledge and an intuitive approach – whereby the HPS 'tunes-in' to the needs, abilities or behaviours of a child, and responds to their cues 'in the moment'.

Reflecting on my experience of supporting Ron and his mum during this procedure, I realised how many things I was seeing on entering the cubicle, as well as how many questions were raised.

At this point in the story, I can see:

- Ron is sweaty and crying. He is showing physical signs of distress. – What can I do? Should I calm him down? Or distract him?
- Ron is having seizures.
- Ron is about to slip out of his mother's hands.
- Ron's mum looks uncomfortable in her physical position, and she is emotionally distressed. How can I support her?

I wonder why:

- The doctor has had three attempts at IV access already. Can we have a break?
- There is no one else here to support the doctor, Ron or his mum.
- There is no additional help to do this procedure safely.
- We are in Ron's cubicle. Could we move this procedure to the treatment room?
- Ron has not been given any local anaesthetic to his skin. Could we use a local anaesthetic if the procedure is repeated?

Part of the HPS's role is to calm the procedural situation in order to keep children relaxed. The HPS is often involved in advocating for space and for breaks for children and families from stressful interventions (HPSET & NAHPS, 2019, 4:5). This can also give other staff (in this case the doctor) a space to stop, reflect and rethink their plan in collaboration with the HPS and other colleagues. It is then important to wait for the right moment until a child is settled, before starting to engage in play, as well as the next steps.

Only once Ron was settled could I pop out of the cubicle and quickly get my distraction box and a guided imagery book. I also collected some animal figures from the playroom as Ron loves animals. Once my resources were in hand, I headed straight back to Ron's bed space.

Dr Trelawny re-enters the cubicle saying the consultant decided to insert a mid-line into Ron's arm. The team are coming with the equipment and the ultrasound machine.

Ron is looking through the distraction box, and interacting with me and mum. He is still having seizures but continues playing. I stay with Ron and mum whilst we wait for the arrival of the medical team.

Mum says she will step out for this procedure as she does not feel she can comfort him or cope herself. I reassure her that I will stay with Ron to support him.

The medical team arrive, and the consultant introduces himself to Ron's mum, explaining what they plan to do.

I notice Ron looking at all the new faces. So I say, "This is the doctor who is going to help us get the special little straw into your arm so we can give you the medicine you need to feel better". This prompts the consultant to say "Hello" directly to Ron. Ron looks over at him but looks away. He pulls his legs close to his chest.

I continue playing using toys from my distraction box. Ron smiles and takes a toy car from my hand tracking it along his bed.

Ron's mum agrees to the mid-line and informs the team that she will be outside and return once the procedure is complete. Then she leaves the cubicle.

That leaves Ron, myself, the consultant, a critical outreach nurse, Dr Trelawny and a staff nurse in the cubicle. The medical team is setting up their sterile equipment. Ron is playing on his bed with me.

As we play, I incorporate instructions about how he needs to sit for the procedure – getting him to wiggle up the bed and sit back in a comfortable position, knowing this will allow him to play whilst being in an appropriate position for the procedure. We are ready.

The consultant re-enters the cubicle, gowned-up and ready to start. He asks the other staff to swaddle Ron in a sheet with one arm out. The nurse begins to pull a sheet around Ron's body.

I speak up, sharing my concerns that I don't feel this is appropriate. Ron may become more distressed if he is restricted under a tight sheet.

At first the team doesn't share my view. They pause and look back to the consultant for instructions. I continue playing, and ask Ron if he could put his arm out, so the doctor can look with his special machine.

Ron refuses.

Part of the HPS's role is advocating for the needs of the children (HPSET & NAHPS 2:1, 4:1, 4:5 2019), e.g. their need for play or how their treatment happens. Whatever the reason, it is hard to speak out during a procedure to ask for a change of plan, even when you know that request is in the best interests of the child (UNICEF, 1989). It is frustrating when you have prepared the child fully and know you can help them cope, only to have the plan changed by other staff members, such as by the suggestion to restrain or re-position them. In these situations, the HPS must be both diplomat and advocate.

Here, Ron is refusing to cooperate with the consultant.

I have to work with him carefully whilst everyone is waiting. The pressure is on! I need to incorporate play to engage and encourage Ron's cooperation. The medical team has other views, but I keep the room light and calm by continuing with my plan. I am ready to explain the benefits of patient engagement, choice during medical interventions and desensitisation of environment, but it is not needed. What happens next proves my professional knowledge and instinct.

I pick a lion figure from my pocket and walk it over to his arm and 'RAWR' really loud.

Ron laughs and I say, "Can you put your arm out for the Lion to look at?"

Ron laughs and relinquishes his tight grip of his arm and lets me place the lion in his hand.

The consultant nods at me, smiles and the nurse holds Ron's arm steady whilst the consultant uses the ultrasound machine to find a strong vein to insert the mid-line.

Ron glances at what they are doing but is distracted by the appearance of a new animal from my pocket. It's a penguin!

So now we have Ron's right hand secure with the nurse and consultant and his left free for play and distraction. Phew! First step complete! With the help of my silly animal impressions, Ron is co-operating without being restrained.

Amongst the elephant impressions and car vs penguin battles, in the midst of invasive procedures, I listened. I watched the room and waited for cues; when would the next step start – in this case, the insertion of a mid-line. Then I juggled immersive play and distraction, thus ensuring the child's safety during the procedure; giving positive reinforcement, whilst keeping his positioning correct; recognising pauses in play which are seizures – or perhaps a show of anxiety? – whilst also observing the medical team and how far through the procedure we all are. A HPS must be an expert in juggling – and not in the way others might expect!

The consultant informs Dr Trelawny he has a suitable vein and prepares to insert the line. I notice there is nothing shielding Ron from the medical team, so I place my distraction book (turned to the animal page) to block his view of the procedure.

The consultant tells Ron they are ready to put in first the local anaesthetic and then the line. I notice Ron is seizing as they start inserting the line. Seconds later Ron immerges from this focal seizure and cries out, but he keeps still and I reassure him that he is doing a great job.

I see he is looking at the animals in the book and I ask him to find a giraffe. He finds the giraffe with his left hand. I ask what noise a giraffe makes; he doesn't know so I make a noise. Ron laughs and says, "That's a monkey noise!"

We continue spotting animals in the book and Ron laughs as I adopt different impressions. He is my focus, yet I can hear that the medical team have successfully placed the mid-line and are now applying the dressing and bandage. Ron is still engrossed in playing on the bed.

I lower the book and Ron looks across at his arm. He points and says, "Is that my special straw Katie?" I reply "Yes it is! You were amazing! I think the Lion helped keep your arm still!" Ron laughs and roars loudly.

The medical team leave the cubical thanking everyone for their help.

There are many elements enabling this procedure to be successful. However, without the professional knowledge and skills of the HPS, this procedure would have been a very different experience for Ron.

Whilst play and distraction did not take away pain or discomfort, they did encourage the child's engagement which led to the procedure being a more positive experience for everyone involved. Advocating for children and young people during medical procedures is complex and can be difficult. Every child and every situation is unique.

I hope in my role as a HPS, my work is valuable not just because of the impact on the experiences of children and their families but also on medical professionals who get to see how the 'magic of play' can have a positive impact on procedural interventions.

References

Healthcare Play Specialist Education Trust and National Association of Health Play Specialists. (2019) *Health Play Specialist Standards of Proficiency Professional Standards.* [Online] Available at: <https://hpset.org.uk/registration-responsibilities/> [Accessed 8 May 2022].

Hubbuck, C. (2009) *Play for Sick Children.* London: Jessica Kingsley Publishers.

Perasso, G., Camurati, G., Morrin, E., Dill, C., Dolidze, K., Clegg, T., Simonelli, I., Lo, H. Y.C., Magione-Standish, A., Pansier, B., Gulyurtlu, S. C., Garone, A. and Rippen, H. (2021) Five Reasons Why Pediatric Settings Should Integrate the Play Specialist and Five Issues in Practice. *Frontiers in Psychology,* 12. Doi: 10.3389/fpsyg.2021.687292

Tonkin, A. ed. (2014) *Play in Healthcare: Using Play to Promote Child Development and Well-being.* Abingdon: Routledge.

UNICEF (1989) *The United Nations Convention on the Rights of the Child.* [Online] Available at: <https://www.unicef.org.uk/what-we-do/un-convention-child-rights/> [Accessed 5 May 2022].

Walker, J. (2006) *Play for Health: Delivering and Auditing Quality in Hospital Play Services.* London: National Association of Hospital Play Staff (NAHPS).

9

A DAY IN THE LIFE OF A HEALTH PLAY SPECIALIST

Katie Collis – Health Play Specialist

The purpose of play in hospital is to provide psychological preparation and support to children who are being seen or cared for by various paediatric professionals who together make up a multidisciplinary healthcare team (MDT). The person whose primary responsibility of the delivery of play in hospital is a health play specialist (HPS), a specifically trained, registered professional who uses play as a therapeutic tool to help and support sick children and young people in healthcare settings. The importance of this work has been recognised as far back as the Platt Report (Ministry of Health, 1959) which was released at a similar time to the groundbreaking work of James and Joyce Robertson. The Robertsons, working with John Bowlby, presented findings that highlighted the specific needs of young children in hospital and the risks they faced there to their social and emotional well-being. Both Robertson and Platt made a strong case for children needing structure and for the richness of play to be woven into their hospital care.

More recently the role and work of the HPS have been described and discussed in greater detail. Hubbuck (2009) suggested that Hugh Jolly's original 1976 description of the HPS still 'succinctly, yet accurately' describes the role of the HPS, while recognising that training and the health service have evolved. In a nutshell, "the play specialist helps the child cope with the experience of being in hospital" (Jolly, 1976, cited in Hubbuck, 2009, p. 35). Following research into the HPS's role, and in an expansion of this early description Perez-Duarte presented an understanding of HPSs as "professional healthcare-workers who advocate for children and use 'playful' methods to improve communication with, and the lived-experience of, children in hospital" (Perez-Duarte, 2022, p. 1). However, the role of the HPS seems to be rather misunderstood within the context of today's MDTs (Perasso et al., 2021). There is also no agreed and established method of practice that is recognised and understood by HPSs and

DOI: 10.4324/9781003255444-12

their colleagues, irrespective of the healthcare setting. This could contribute to the role of the HPS being better understood – and their skills used as well as possible – in supporting children and young people throughout their hospital experiences.

Everyday working as a HPS is different. This is part of the joy of the job! Walking into the unexpected – as well as the occasional planned and expected engagements – with children and young people and their families, is motivating and challenging. There are always different and new priorities to juggle.

Within this chapter my intention is to give an insight into the daily work of the HPS and how this looks from the point of view of the practitioner, and what it feels like with some sense of events happening 'in real time'. This will be achieved by the inclusion of a central case study and my first-hand reflections of how time was managed and priorities reshuffled throughout the day to ensure the needs of patients and expectations of the MDT were met.

Ana was brought to my attention by a member of nursing staff just after handover. The handover was brief, but it was explained that the patient was anxious and would require some support.

I had other children who required some preparation for surgery and general anaesthetics. After preparing these other patients, I went to speak to Ana.

Ana and her mum explained to me that Ana had experienced some traumatic health experiences in the past – particularly around blood tests.

I purposefully spent some time with Ana and her mum as I felt it was important for them both to feel reassured and supported at this time. I provided Ana with some play resources – some colouring of her favourite things and some games to play with her mum – reassuring them that I would return later in the morning to check-in and see how they were.

Some HPS colleagues find it helpful to plan their day, hour by hour, but others find this too constraining. My personal preference is to highlight patients on the paperwork from the nursing handover, followed by writing a list of other tasks and appointments as aims to meet throughout the day. This way there is a certain degree of flexibility as well as planning for the resources which may be needed – ideally these toys, activities and craft materials, as well as more specialised items for preparation and distraction, are all easily accessible and ready to grab at a moment's notice. Our team have 'grab and go' boxes of preparation resources for different medical procedures, as well as for different types of more general play. This way, when arranging sessions for children, it is easier to meet children's requests, needs and preferences and setting-up takes less time.

It was apparent from the nursing handover at the start of the day that there were a number of patients who may require the support of a HPS – and that I was the only HPS on duty (with a Health Play Assistant (HPA) colleague). The initial priority was to attend to the children who would be going to theatre imminently and prepare them for their surgery – there were six children on the morning list. It has been recognised that adequate pre-operative information is essential to child and their parents and that preparation for surgery can mean the patient is less stressed and may recover quicker (RCN, 2020). On my arrival at work on any given day, it is always a priority to establish how may children are likely to need this support and input.

The next priority was to make contact with the patients who had been in for an extended amount of time. At that time, the ward had three babies and one toddler as long-term patients. It is generally acknowledged that children are likely to suffer some degree of emotional disturbance from prolonged or repeated hospital admission (Bonn, 1994). However, children being able to understand their experiences, facilitated by 'knowledgeable others', assist them with the negotiating and problem solving that such an experience may bring (Palaiologou, 2013). That knowledgeable other person is often the HPS who, by their training and skill in working with children in hospitals, is able to scaffold the learning and guide the patient towards a greater understanding of their situation.

A little while later, during a session with another patient, I was informed that Ana required a blood test and the insertion of a cannula ahead of an MRI later on, and I was asked to assist and support her with this.

When I asked when this would be, the nurse responded by saying, "Well, ideally now".

I challenged this and asked if there was time for some local anaesthetic cream to be applied as I was aware of Ana's previous negative experiences and wanted to try to improve today's medical interventions as much as possible.

I explained I would be there as soon as I could. This was agreed but perhaps – I felt – with a little resistance to the way I was advocating for Ana.

As well as the surgical list and long-term patients there were – like on so many other General Medical wards – other recently admitted children who potentially needed support, mostly from an HPS although some activities could be undertaken by a HPA, and these were delegated accordingly. This is the reality of the HPS's role where multiple patients require a range of input, often at similar times due to the nature of covering more than one paediatric area. The need to continuously reassess priorities throughout the day, and respond appropriately, efficiently and effectively, is a skill that the HPS, as an autonomous professional who exercises their own professional judgement, learns and develops throughout their training and career. This aspect of the role is outlined in items 4 and 9 of the HPSET Standards of Proficiency (HPSET, 2019). This states that as trained, registered practitioners, HPSs should "be able to assess a professional situation ... and to act within your professional scope of practise at all times" (4.1) and to "be able to contribute effectively to work undertaken as part of a professional team" (9.4).

A positive part of working as a team made up of both HPSs and HPAs (and additionally in some settings, volunteers) is that when that team works well together, the duties of the day are planned and prioritised (and then re-prioritised), and much of the general play, developmental play parental and/or sibling support, can be shared with colleagues, leaving the more specialised requirements to the HPS. In hospitals or ward areas where there is not this variety of roles within a team, where HPSs are 'lone workers' or where staff sickness or leave does not warrant additional cover, the HPS must further try to prioritise the tasks of the day to cover and provide for children and families considered to be most in need

During the day, whilst waiting to continue assisting Ana, there were other varied requests and pulls on my working day. These included:

- Five children who required support with invasive procedures – amounting to five distractions including one preparation and play session
- Being called by a physiotherapy colleague requesting support for a child's outpatient splint fitting
- A request for a member of the play team to 'just sit with the patient' while the parent went home to get fresh clothes (this type of request increases as inpatient ward's struggle with being short of staff)
- And lastly (but by no means least) there were administrative tasks to be done alongside the practical 'patient-facing' work – responding to referrals, calling referrers to clarify details, preparation for a one-off celebration week, plus responding to emails

---

From previous encounters, I had established that Ana would be able to cope with her MRI scan. I had prepared her for the scan using a Lego model and photo book, and we agreed that she would attend the radiology department with her parents.

The MRI scan revealed Ana had a brain tumour. The doctors requested that I spend time with Ana whilst they discussed the results with her parents, which I did, and we completed a craft activity together. Upon their return, Ana's parents asked me to stay as they spoke with her so I can help her understand what was happening, ensuring terminology was understood and that the next steps in her journey were clear for her.

Ana was understandably upset and anxious with the details of her diagnosis, and I spent some time supporting her and her parents. We then played a board game all together which I felt helped to 'ground' the family after such a distressing day. Shortly afterwards, as I was completing my shift, Ana was transferred to a specialist hospital for further care.

> As they left, I made a telephone call to the HPS team at the specialist hospital to handover to them and communicate the work Ana and I had done together. This also provided an opportunity to discuss her previous negative experiences and main anxiety triggers. My work with Ana and her family – stretching through the whole day – was now complete.

Reflecting back, this day was busy and demanding, but not unusual. Everyday working as a HPS is varied, sometimes to the point of being unpredictable, and a requirement of the job is the ability to adapt, plan and prioritise as you go. Working with Ana and her family was highly rewarding and also a challenge that required to be 'on-call' *for* Ana throughout the day, yet not necessarily *with* her for the whole time. In the 'in-between' times, it was necessary to return to the in-patient and day-case wards and to attend to children in those areas who were also in need of support.

This work relies on good communication between the HPS and their multidisciplinary team colleagues. It also requires resources that are accessible and plentiful since leaving children waiting for procedures means leaving them with whatever activities are going to make their wait manageable. Being able to offer them a variety of activities – sometimes multiple times throughout the day – should keep boredom, anxiety and disruption to a minimum as they await procedures, examinations and discussions with healthcare professionals.

During the day some important work was done. It is important to acknowledge, however, that not everything was completed. I was unable to support a child in another ward. Timing collided with Ana's procedure and the ward staff did not wait until I was available. It is not unusual for this to happen and staff there will assess whether they feel a child will cope without play support. The reality is that if ward teams waited for me on every occasion, my changing workload would soon cause a backlog with their patients. While it is not ideal, it is always possible to offer post-procedural play, particularly if a child is known to require future interventions. Similarly, three of the long-term patients had a shorter session than normal with a HPA, but on less demanding days, it would be possible to spend longer with each of them, following their play programme and trying to ensure that their developmental goals were being met. Finally, in the course of the day, it was not possible to undertake any administrative tasks, beyond writing in children's healthcare notes, outlining the play provision they had received and a quick email check. My HPA colleague undertook some preparation for *Play in Hospital Week* (an annual celebration in the UK of the work and provision of hospital play teams), planning and piecing together a wall display and timetable of activities. These are all important elements of the HPS role but can be time-consuming and sometimes lose out to the immediate demands of the HPS's patient-facing work.

In spite of these demands and pressures, on reflection, it is clear that the HPSs work with children and their families and make a considerable difference to their experiences of being in hospital. One of the biggest challenges is having to regularly re-evaluate throughout each day to ensure children's needs are best met. This sometime includes seeking support from colleagues and the reallocation of the work. The work requires a very particular mix of professional judgement – understanding the complexity of clinical procedures, examinations and environments, recognising and responding to children's developmental and emotional needs and managing the stresses and unpredictability of the hospital environment.

To be a HPS also requires a significant amount of personal and professional resilience. It is challenging working with very sick or distressed children, and it is equally necessary to stay both calm 'in the moment' whilst processing each encounter as it happens. The ways we each manage this balancing act will be very individualised, but some key elements include good teamwork, effective communication, access to support or supervision at work and cultivating a good work-life balance.

Being a HPS is brilliant. Not easy – and certainly not 'just playing all day' – but to do this work is rewarding and challenging, effortful and joyful – all in fairly equal measure.

References

Bonn, M. (1994) The effects of hospitalisation on children: A review. *Curationis* 17 (2) pp. 20–24

HPSET (2019) *Health Play Specialist Standards of Proficiency Professional Standards* [Online] Health Play Specialist Education Trust and National Association of Health Play Specialists. Available from: <https://hpset.org.uk/HPSET_ps.pdf> [Accessed 3 August 2022]

Hubbuck, C. (2009) *Play for Sick Children: Play Specialists in Hospitals and Beyond*. London. Jessica Kingsley Publishers

Jolly, H. (1976) Why children must be able to play in hospital. *The Times*, 21 April.

Ministry of Health (1959) *The Welfare of Children in Hospital, The Platt Report)*. London: HMSO

Palaiologou, I. (ed.) (2013) *The Early Years Foundation Stage: Theory and Practice*. 2nd Edition. London: Sage Publications

Perasso, G., Camurati, G., Morrin, E., Dill, C., Dolidze, K., Clegg, T., Simonelli, I., Lo, H., Magione-Standish, A., Pansier, B., Gulyurtlu, S., Garone, A. & Rippen, H. (2021) Five reasons why pediatric settings should integrate the play specialist and five issues in practice. *Frontiers in Psychology* 12. Doi: 10.3389/Fpsyg.2021.687292

Perez-Duarte, P. (2022) How to communicate with children according to Health Play Specialists in the United Kingdom: A qualitative study. *Journal of Child Health Care* [Online] Available from: <https://journals.sagepub.com/doi/pdf/10.1177/13674935221109113> [Accessed 12 August 2022]

RCN (2020) *Day Surgery for Children and Young People: RCN Guidance*. London: Royal College of Nursing

Robertson, J. & Robertson, J. (1971) Young children in brief separation: A fresh look *Psychoanalytic Study of the Child* 26, pp. 264–315

10

TEENAGERS IN HOSPITAL

Are they the forgotten age?

*Nicky Everett – Senior Lecturer
and Health Play Specialist*

Within any NHS Hospital the staff will encounter people from all walks of life, all with different cultural backgrounds, upbringings, different ethnicities and genders, and importantly for this chapter, a variety of age groups.

When a child is particularly unwell, they are likely to be admitted to hospital and they will be treated in a paediatric ward or outpatient department. During this admission, children will be looked after by trained and qualified paediatric staff. As for adults, they will be admitted to a specific or specialised adult unit, and this will be staffed with trained and qualified adult nurses, doctors, physiotherapists, dieticians, etc. However, if you are a teenager/adolescent, aged between 13 and 18 years where do you go? This age group does not sit comfortably within paediatrics, as teenagers do not really see themselves as children anymore, but in the same context they are not quite adults either. There seems to be a gap in the research around the needs of adolescents in hospital (Blumberg & Devlin, 2006), so this chapter will examine life for teenagers within a hospital setting and explore where they fit in, during a stressful and unsettling time in their life, even prior to a hospital admission.

What is adolescence?

Adolescence is the transition period between childhood and adulthood. Between the ages of 9 and 21 years, girls and boys start out as children, mentally and physically, and end the phase as adults (Hopkins, 2014). Rupp and Yantis (2021) suggest adolescence is divided into three stages, early (ages 12–14), middle (ages 15–17) and late (ages 18–21). During these stages each young person will develop and mature at their own rate. Often this phase is associated with turbulence ... risk taking, rebelling, seeking independence and

DOI: 10.4324/9781003255444-13

pushing boundaries. Arain et al. (2013, p. 451) suggest, "Adolescence is one of the most dynamic events of human growth and development, second only to infancy in terms of the rate of developmental changes that can occur within the brain". Over the past 25 years, through Magnetic Resonance Imaging (MRI) there has been extensive research around the adolescent brain (Arain et al., 2013) examining how within this stage the brain is still 'under construction'. When thinking about a hospital admission, this can have implications for rehabilitation and intervention (Costandi, 2014). Development does not stop at childhood it continues into adolescence and we continue to change in both predictable and unpredictable ways throughout our lifetime, even into old age (Kuther, 2019).

Erik Erikson, a developmental psychologist, maintained that personality develops in a predetermined order through eight stages of psychosocial development, from infancy to adulthood (Mercer, 2018). Through the transitional years Erikson examined crisis points that an adolescent may encounter which they must face and resolve (Keenan et al., 2016). This stage he labelled as a period where young people entered a crisis point of *Identity v Confusion* as adolescents strive to discover who they are. Erikson believed that the formation of identity and a sense of self was one of the most important conflicts people face (Walker & Horner, 2020). Alongside this he examined the potentially unfavourable outcomes for young people during this time, which he identified as a young person having some confusion over who and what one really is (Sacco, 2013). Throughout this adolescent period, young people are trying to gain more independence within their life away from their main caregivers, their bodies are changing, friendships are often being tested, suddenly they must start thinking about their future, drugs and/or alcohol may be introduced and there may be relationships developing. Combine all of this with a hospital admission or a diagnosis that could mean extensive periods of time spent in hospital, and a young person may suddenly find themselves in turmoil.

Adolescents in hospital

Entering a hospital, can be a scary and daunting time, which carries a huge amount of uncertainty, regardless of the patient's age. As identified by Erikson, the potential confusion within the adolescence stage could mean that being admitted to hospital may have a huge impact on how they deal with certain situations, as some young people can often give the impression of possessing adult logic and coping skills (Blumberg & Devlin, 2006), when in reality, that is not always the case. An admission could result in a young person becoming more vulnerable and suddenly feeling they have lost any independence they had, becoming more reliant on their caregivers than usual and with increased time in hospital, friendships or relationships may start to decline which can have a real impact on a young person's mental health.

PERSONAL REFLECTION

I worked as a youth support coordinator on a Teenage Cancer Unit for just over eight years. When a young person was initially diagnosed, they were often surrounded by friends coming to visit them on the ward, but as time went on these friendships seemed to dwindle and the young person in hospital then spent a lot of time watching their friends enjoying life through social media. However, on the flip side, some young people would ask their friends not to visit, and slowly pull away. This was a result of how they felt about themselves and their appearance; they felt they had changed and no longer looked the same as they did. This was often down to their hair loss or because they had gained weight due to the impact of steroid treatment. On the other hand, some young people needed support with their weight loss and calorie intake, so they had a nasal gastric (NG) tube fitted, which is taped to their cheek, and they didn't want their friends to see this, becoming very self-conscious. I was often told by the female patients that the worst part of their diagnosis was their hair loss, and the build-up to this happening brought about more stress than the treatment itself.

Lefevre (2010) discussed how professionals should be communicating with young people. She explains that some older young people can find discussing private and sensitive issues uncomfortable or embarrassing, with the adolescent years being a time of heightened self-consciousness. Young people have expressed how when speaking to professionals they want that individual to be confident in discussing topics around such things as sexual health, mental health, substance misuse or relationships (Lefevre, 2010), i.e., the issues that young people often face during adolescence. In respect of this, being admitted to a unit that is not specifically for adolescents can cause further stress and anxieties.

Across the UK, wards and departments that are explicitly for adolescents do not exist. This is with the exception of those attending a Teenage Oncology Ward, where with help and funding from The Teenage Cancer Trust (a body external to the NHS), designated units and staff are available for teenagers during their cancer treatment. The Teenage Cancer Trust (2021) states: "Our 28 specialist units within NHS hospitals bring young people aged between 13 and 24 together, to be treated by teenage cancer experts in a place designed just for them".

PERSONAL REFLECTION

These teenage specific wards give young people a place to be themselves alongside other young people of a similar age. They have Day Rooms to hang out in, with Sky TV, gaming stations, pool tables, comfy chairs and an amazing juke box (funded by the Teenage Cancer Trust). They also have a Youth

Support Coordinator on the unit who is there to support and make the hospital feel a little less scary. They provide the opportunity to socialise and meet other patients on the ward, in a space that is not as clinical, but more like a youth club. Through taking time to chat, playing cards or just having breakfast with the young people in a relaxed way, it was clear to me that they felt able to talk more freely about their concerns, worries regarding treatment and general issues concerning their future.

Based on my experience, having separate wards with staff skilled in working with adolescents enhances the experience for these young people, creating more of a therapeutic environment, which is beneficial for all of those admitted (Macfarlane & Blum, 2001). However, Macfarlane and Blum (2001) write that the need for this is difficult to prove and there have been no controlled studies undertaken to show such an impact; this was, however, over 20 years ago and although a lot has changed in this time, little has been done to fill this void in the research.

For the purpose of this chapter, I spoke to four young adults who were all admitted and treated in hospital during their adolescent years. I asked them to tell me how it made them feel when they were admitted to a children's ward during their time in hospital while undergoing treatment. These are their responses ...

RESPONSE A – "It just made me feel more different than I already felt. I almost felt babied, and the staff were lovely, but you could tell they were not used to looking after a 17-year-old. It was hard not having people to chat to who understood what is was like being a young adult in hospital".

RESPONSE B – "Having the teenage ward was amazing and made the whole experience so much easier. I will always be really grateful for that ward".

RESPONSE C – "Glad we had the ward ##, we could all relate to each other without having to start explaining how we felt or what we were going through, and no one felt sorry for each other".

RESPONSE D – "I found that the day started a lot earlier than the teenage ward, which was annoying as I could not get as much sleep due to staying up later. Also, there was no place to go during the day but the playroom, which was full of toys for the younger kids and not much for me to do. The play team who came round also only catered for the younger kids. I felt out of place being surrounded by kids much younger than me, whereas when there are teenagers around it gives you the chance to talk to them, make friends and share with them what you're going through".

In theory the Health Play Specialist (HPS) role will work with children and young people from 0 to 18 years, but from my own experience and from speaking to others, this can be a challenging balance. Some wards do try and provide a specific teen area for them to 'hang out' in, away from the playroom. However, on discussion with fellow HPS staff this room will often be used for meetings or what is often labelled 'The Bad News Room':

RESPONSE 1 – Southern England
"We have no separate space for teens ☹. I think we do have resources for them, but limited and contained to their own bedspace.
Teens are mixed in with all ages in the bay".

RESPONSE 2 – West Midlands
"On our children's wards we don't have a specific area for teens, they are with all ages".

RESPONSE 3 – Southwest
"Our teenagers end up mixed in with all ages in the bay. We lost our teenage room as it was needed to be used for other things".

Play is often seen as something that only children engage in (Powell, 2022). Some of the HPS staff above also commented on how teenage engagement was not always great from the young people during their time on the ward "… I am happy working with teenagers. However, sometimes they just want to be on their phones, have a DVD or play on the Nintendo Switch" (Response 3 – Southwest). However, linking this to the comments made by the young people it appears they do not always feel comfortable engaging while on a 'children's ward' surrounded by children and toys. Young people may not acknowledge that they still want to play and may not recognise their engagement as play. However, through play teenagers continue to develop, which enhances their communication, cooperation and negotiation skills (Whitaker & Tonkin, 2021).

PERSONAL REFLECTION

I was often asked how I enjoyed working with teenagers, "are they not just in bed all day" and "when they are awake are they not just really stroppy". No, they are not always, would be my response! Play was a big part of my role as a YSC, a game of cards (usually Shit Head), nibbles and a hot chocolate, got most teenagers out of bed. This gave me the opportunity to engage with them in a way that did not feel forced. While playing cards, you do not need to look at each other. You don't always have to talk either, but often lots of talking did happen and through play this was a safe place to do so. Young people who find it hard to share their feelings or concerns will often talk more when they are relaxed and feeling like they are choosing to have that conversation, as opposed to being in a consultation style planned meeting, which happened often for these young people. So, in answer to the initial question, I loved my job.

For a young person during these adolescent years and from my own personal work experience, having access to a designated young person's ward is so important, for their own well-being and mental health. Having the opportunity to access a ward or unit with professionals who understand you is important for us all, so why should it be any different for teenagers?

References

Arain, M., Haque, M., Johal, L., Mathur, P., Nel, W., Rais, A., Sandhu, R. and Sharma, S. (2013) Maturation of the Adolescent Brain. *Neuro Psychiatric Disease and Treatment*, 9 (9), pp. 449–461.

Blumberg, R. and Devlin, A.S. (2006) Design Issues in Hospitals: The Adolescent Client. *Environment and Behavior*, 38 (3), pp. 293–317.

Costandi, M. (2014) *Adolescent Brain Development*. [Online] Available from: https://thinkneuroscience.wordpress.com/2014/01/22/adolescent-brain-development/ [Accessed 27 January 2022].

Hopkins, J.R. (2014) *Adolescence*. London: Academic Press.

Keenan, T., Evans, S. and Crowley, K. (2016) *An Introduction to Child Development*, 3rd Edition. London: SAGE.

Kuther, T. (2019) *Lifespan Development Lives in Context*. California: SAGE.

Lefevre, M. (2010) *Communicating with Children and Young People*. Bristol: Policy Press.

Macfarlane, A. and Blum, R. (2001) Do We Need Specialist Adolescent Units in Hospitals? *BMJ*, 322 (7292), pp. 941–942.

Mercer, J. (2018) *Child Development: Concepts & Theories*. London: SAGE.

Powell, S. (2022) *Playtime: Is it time we took 'play' more seriously? BBC News*, 13 January 2022. [Online] Available from: https://www.bbc.co.uk/news/entertainment-arts-59950823 [Accessed 15 June 2022].

Rupp, R. and Yantis, E. (2021). Adolescent Medicine. In: Niebuhr. V. and Urbani, M. *Core Concepts of Pediatrics. An Online Resource for Residents and Medical Students*. 2nd Edition. The University of Texas Medical Branch. [Online] Available from: https://www.utmb.edu/pedi_ed/CoreV2/Adolescent/Adolescent.html [Accessed 27 January 2022].

Sacco, R. (2013). Re-Envisaging the Eight Developmental Stages of Erik Erikson: The Fibonacci Life-Chart Method (FLCM). *Journal of Educational and Developmental Psychology*, 3 (1), pp. 140–146.

Teenage Cancer Trust (2021). *Youth Support Coordinators*. [Online] Available from: https://www.teenagecancertrust.org [Accessed 15 June 2022].

Walker, J. and Horner, N. (2020). *Social Work and Human Development*, 6th Edition. London: SAGE.

Whitaker, J. and Tonkin, A. (2021). *Play for Health across the Lifespan*. Abingdon: Routledge.

11

SPECIALISED PLAY IN THE HOSPITAL SETTING

Susan Fairclough – Managerial and Professional Lead for Therapeutic and Specialised Play Service, Youth Service Manager and Events Lead

This chapter highlights the vital and essential role of the qualified and registered health play specialist (HPS). Specialised play in hospital and the healthcare setting is explained, and various techniques utilised by the HPS to help children and young people are examined. There is also a discussion of the use of specialised play in preparing and minimising the effects of illness and hospitalisation for children of all ages, abilities and needs. Finally, there is an examination of how this helps to provide a positive experience for the patient and family through their hospital and healthcare journey.

The importance of play

Play is an essential foundation and a vital part of every child's life. It helps normal growth and development enabling a child or young person to develop physically, intellectually, emotionally, socially and verbally. Through play, children acquire knowledge and learn new skills that prepare them to cope with the world around them (Whitebread, 2012). Play is a rich learning medium that allows children and young people of all ages and abilities to communicate. Play enables children and young people to learn whilst involved in an activity or recreational activity. Through play, children absorb information which then becomes part of their knowledge, skills and development.

Play is fun and it can present as a method to assess children's development, how they cooperate, participate and understand. In a hospital setting, many assessments and observations use various methods of play and activities, as play is a universal language and is inclusive for all. Play forms a critical part in implementing public health agendas and accident prevention programmes, influencing children's understanding and behaviour (Fairclough and Bennett, 2021).

DOI: 10.4324/9781003255444-14

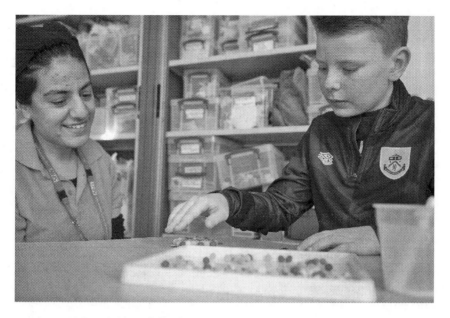

FIGURE 11.1 Creativity with beads.

Communicating healthy messages and engaging children and young people in fun and enjoyable activities to promote healthy behaviours is key, as well as facilitating recovery from illness and injury.

It is important to understand and acknowledge the essential role play has in the foundation of development, learning and understanding that will equip children and young people throughout their lives (Figure 11.1).

The place of specialised play in the health play specialist's role

In 1959 the Platt Report acknowledged that the provision of play in healthcare settings is an important element in meeting the child and young person's holistic needs (Ministry of Health, 1959). From this, the National Association for the Welfare of Children in Hospital (NAWCH, now named Action for Sick Children) was formed. In 1975, formalisation of the provision of play in hospital led to the establishment of the National Association of Health Play Specialists (NAHPS). NAHPS championed the change in culture and attitude towards the need for play provision in children's health services and drove the process of professionalisation of the HPS role. This position is now an established part of children and young people's healthcare teams, and the importance of play continues to feature across contemporary child health policies (Royal College of Paediatrics and Child Health, 2019).

In today's health service, HPSs have a fundamental role within all multidisciplinary teams (MDT) in the holistic care and support of the physical and mental health and well-being of children and young people in hospital and healthcare settings. They are an integral part of the MDT, providing developmental and therapeutic play to help patients in hospital from an appointment or admission through to discharge and possible readmission due to long-term conditions or treatments. HPSs also provide specialised play, helping with the psychological, emotional and physical aspects of preparation for patients attending hospital appointments and being admitted for treatments, procedures and surgery. They liaise closely with the other health professionals to provide support and information, introducing this through a variety of specialised play activities, preparation clinics and therapeutic play sessions.

With play as the central function of their role, and as integral members of the multidisciplinary healthcare team, the work of HPSs positively enhances the quality of care provided for children and young people (Walker, 2006). HPSs are involved in the design and delivery of play services and undertake a range of activities and interventions that ensure play forms a part of every child's healthcare experience. In play teams, HPSs may work alongside play leaders, play assistants or playworkers, colleagues who have not undertaken the specific HPS training but who contribute to the provision of general, developmental play for children in a hospital setting.

All HPSs are qualified, trained and experienced professionals who work within paediatric teams. To use the title, they must have completed the Healthcare Play Specialism for Sick Children FDA (Foundation or Full Degree Course). They are then registered and must re-register annually with the Health Play Specialist Education Trust (HPSET). Registered HPSs work in accordance with the Code of Professional Conduct and Standards for Professional Practice as set out by HPSET.

Many HPSs also have additional qualifications, up to and including degree-level training in Early Childhood Studies, Playwork, Nursery Nursing (NNEB) or other relevant childcare qualification. Based on their training, the HPS is equipped to provide developmental, therapeutic and specialised play for hospitalised children and young people. They help the patients to prepare for hospital or the healthcare environment via patient referrals, pre-admission work, inpatient work, specific preparation for treatments, procedures, surgery, distraction and diversionary play plus post-procedural play interventions. Many HPSs undertake individual patient referrals besides the ward/department patients and ward activity. With experience and knowledge gained 'on the job' they can assist children and young people to help desensitisation from hospital phobias and fears, where a trusting therapeutic relationship is deepened through play (Kool and Lawver, 2010). All children staying in hospital should have daily access to a qualified and registered HPS and, while the use of play techniques should be used across the MDT, HPSs take a lead in modelling playful techniques that other staff can adopt in their practice (Department of Health, 2003; Walker, 2006).

What is specialised play?

Play can reduce the psychological trauma of hospitalisation and is the vehicle through which children express and interact (Jolley, 2007). The function of specialised play is to help children and young people to cope with frightening and stressful situations, and to communicate emotions, fears, thoughts and experiences. This is particularly important for children and young people with illness or injury. Through specialised play interventions aimed at the individual child's age and cognitive development level, children and young people can learn why they are attending or staying in hospital, what is going to happen to them and what they will observe, hear and feel in a safe learning environment.

Saile et al. (1988) described psychological preparation as being any planned strategy which is used by a professional or trained helper with the purpose of reducing anxiety related to medical procedures, decreasing pain, accelerating the healing process and making it possible for the child or young person to cope adequately with the procedure. Fear of the unknown, fear of physical harm and pain, loss of control and identity, uncertainty about what is expected of them and separation from security and family routine are identified by Visintainer and Wolfer (1975) as the five key potential threats to a child on admission to hospital.

Through specialised play the HPS helps children and young people to understand many aspects of their healthcare journey and gain information and be educated about their treatment and care. For a child or young person to understand what is happening to them and to be able to ask questions gives them some control when visiting or being admitted to hospital.

Specialised preparation and information-giving – including any visuals, tools or equipment – only need to be basic but they offer simple, clear explanations so that children or young people can understand and ask questions. The HPS liaises closely with parents or carers and refers to healthcare teams for further information if required. Since a child's conception of illness and hospital in the most important factor in determining how well the child will cope (Carson et al., 1992), any specialised play preparation is adjusted by the HPS to suit each individual child or young person whose personality and past experiences may influence their reaction to the hospital and their understanding of procedures.

The HPS may not be the first person to inform a child they are having a procedure, treatment or surgery but they may be the key person who explains the procedure at the child or young person's pace, age and cognitive development level for them to understand. This in turn can assist with a child's informed consent and greater parental understanding of the hospital experience. Preparing children through specialised play preparation sessions and activities is a natural and more creative way to inform them about what will happen to them, who they will meet, what they will observe and experience during their visit or stay in hospital.

Being able to build a rapport and establish a relationship of trust with individual patients is fundamental to the work carried out by HPSs (Hubbuck, 2009).

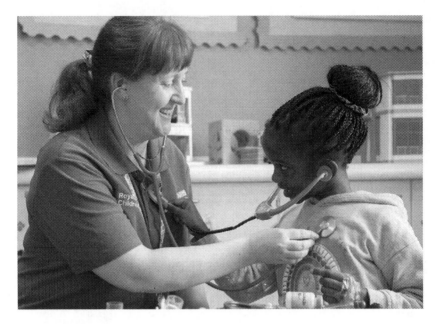

FIGURE 11.2 Preparation work – child and HPS playing with stethoscopes.

They use a variety of specialised resources and activities including role play, various visuals, iPad or tablet, photos and video recordings, preparation apps, models, dolls, photographs, books, jigsaws, auditory recordings, pretend equipment and real equipment. The combination of these resources and tools may be bespoke for individual patients and families. By using these various methods and techniques the HPS helps the children and young people to understand and cope with their plan of treatment, to live with their illnesses, to adapt to their health issues and to move towards recovery (Figure 11.2).

In the next part of this chapter, the focus is on some specific areas of specialised play that are part of the HPS's role with children and young people in a hospital setting. These sections will distinguish between preparation, imaginative hospital role play, basic desensitisation and individual patient referrals and will consider how this work is resourced and delivered.

Preparation

It has long been recognised that children and young people benefit tremendously from preparation and support before hospitalisation (Eiser, 1990; Glasper and Thompson, 1993; Robertson, 1995; While, 1994). This recognition is supported in a number of studies (Adams et al., 1991; Bielby, 1984), which demonstrate that children who receive some type of pre-admission preparation cope much better with hospitalisation, have fewer behavioural problems after discharge, spend less time as an inpatient and return to school more quickly. When a child is admitted in an emergency, time for preparation is extremely limited. Children are often unsure of what is going to happen and may have some additional worries. However, whether it is a planned admission or emergency admission, children and young people respond better when they are supplied with basic information about what is going to happen to them (Ivory, 1998). Play support and age and developmentally appropriate explanations are important to alleviate as much trauma and anxiety as possible.

It is important for children and young people being prepared for admission to hospital that they are empowered to express their views and those views should be heard and respected. If they are unable to communicate their views due to their age or ability, it is important to assess the child's feelings, expressions, body language and any verbal communication and also to liaise closely with their parents or carers to assist with their communication and needs.

The aim of preparation for procedures by the HPS is to help children and young people understand their illness, condition and treatment. It also presents an opportunity to correct any misconceptions they may have. HPSs meet many children and young people who have been previously traumatised and who are now distressed by medical and nursing actions. Through preparation they aim to prevent distress developing at the initial encounter and for children to experience hospital care as positively as possible. Studies by Vessey and Mahon (1990) and Gilman and Frauman (1987) also found play preparation to have great value for children, especially those with a chronic illness. Good preparation – these studies suggest – may result in a happier child who is likely to recover physically from illness more quickly and, therefore, spend less time in hospital. HPSs practice from a position which acknowledges that an informed child is a less vulnerable child and feeling able to cope encourages cooperation (Heiney, 1991) (Figure 11.3).

Preparation through play seeks to improve the child or young person's ability to cope with the healthcare setting. It also may assist informed consent and communication and give space for a rapport and trust to be created between the HPS and the child or young person.

Using various resources and methods to prepare a child or young person is of an important and central aspect of the HPS's role and ideally is done before any procedure or treatment is carried out.

Preparation can take many forms and provides support for a child or young person throughout the various stages of planned admission, these include:

- Pre-Admission – HPS input may happen during specific clinics or appointments for individual children. This may include a tour of the ward or operating theatre areas of the hospital.
- Patient Referral – Specific requests may be made for HPS input prior to admission. (These will be discussed later in the chapter.)
- Appointment Stage – Sometimes decisions or suggestions of hospital admission for treatment or surgery are made during a child's outpatient appointment and input or support is sought from the HPS.

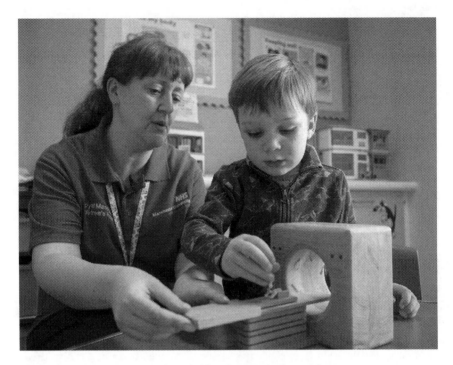

FIGURE 11.3 Preparation work – child and HPS playing with a toy scanner.

- Admission Stage – HPSs may work with children a considerable amount and on numerous occasions during their admission to hospital, to prepare them for each procedure they face, to explain any changes during the course of their treatment or to keep enhancing their understanding of their condition and its treatment.
- Involvement in the procedure following specialised preparation using distraction or diversional play activities. This procedural involvement following the provision of preparation through play is often the ideal scenario for the HPS.
- Post-procedural Play – Here, the HPS returns to the child after their procedure to 'check-in' with them, to informally assess their emotional well-being, to ensure they can ask questions and seek further information as needed and to continue to maintain a relationship of trust that has the potential to be damaged during stressful procedures.

In the *National Service Framework for Children* (2003), the Department of Health describes the type of information that is required, stating that children, young people and parents need "valid, relevant, accurate up to date and easy accessible information that is appropriate to their level of understanding" (Department of Health, 2003, p. 17).

Hospital role play and imaginative play

Gaining the trust of a child enables the HPS and other health professionals to observe their reactions to their hospital experiences and help them cope with any fears, worries and anxieties. Some children or young people do not necessarily show signs of any fear or anxiety, although they still want to be kept informed about what is going to happen to them, when and why and have the opportunity to ask questions.

Hospital play sessions that include aspects of role or imaginary play should take place in a non-clinical environment where the child can feel reassured that no painful procedures or any nursing or medical interventions or treatments are going to take place. Through imaginary and pretend play – play which involves interacting and playing with clinical equipment while supervised, as well as pretend and toy equipment (e.g. doctors/medical sets) – children can be prepared for a variety of treatments, procedures and surgery including having a blood test, observations, having scans, through to having surgery and transplants and so on. By playing in this way children can gain familiarity with medical procedures, equipment and language, ask questions and receive answers that will correct any misinformation or misconceptions (Figure 11.4).

The various types of resources used by HPSs to encourage imaginary, pretend or hospital role play include:

• Pictorial information and diagrams to explain equipment or procedures.
• Dolls and models with medical intravenous lines and tubes.
• Model Hospital sets (including branded sets by PlayMobil, Lego and Happyland).

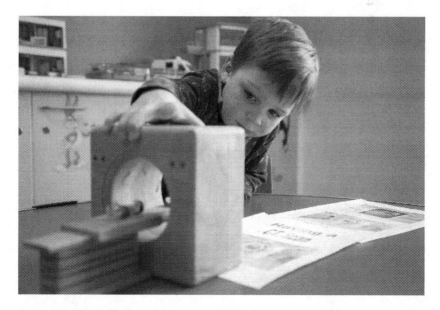

FIGURE 11.4 Specialised equipment – child free-playing with a toy scanner.

- Hospital books – This may include 'social story' type books showing photographs of different stages from hospital admission to discharge, including the hospital environment, clinical surroundings, details of procedures and treatments and health professionals.
- Models of equipment and ways of explaining details of procedures, including audible sounds, e.g. for X-ray and scan machines.
- Dressing up play – Some hospitals can produce healthcare professional's uniforms in child sized versions.
- Technology – iPads/Tablets, including videos, recordings, photographs and Apps explaining treatments and procedures aimed at the child or young person's age and developmental level.

Basic desensitisation

This can be a lengthy process during which a child or young person is subjected to controlled exposure of an object or a situation that causes them some anxiety or fear. The technique involves detailed planning and constant monitoring and must be carried out under qualified and trained professional supervision. Some HPSs offer basic desensitisation, which may take place during specialised play sessions, but most would refer to the psychology team – if they are not already involved – as required.

There are some important things to remember when working with children or young people with specific needs, fears or anxieties in the hospital setting:

- Be honest.
- Use language that is appropriate to a child's age and developmental ability.
- Find out how the child or young person communicates. Do they have any additional needs? Do they use Makaton, signing or symbols to aid communication?
- What are their previous hospital experiences? How do they tell you that these have impacted them? What would they like to understand better or explore?
- Use the correct terms for medical equipment to avoid confusion. Use real names or terms that they will hear and explain what they mean.
- Stay calm and relaxed to instil confidence and reassure the child and family.
- Be aware that the child or young person may not necessarily be fearful of the procedure itself but may be worried about the implications. With an intimate invasive procedure, they may feel embarrassed during the procedure or may be anxious about receiving the result.
- Consider timing when undertaking preparation or desensitisation sessions.
- Always look for non-verbal clues that the child is anxious or is no longer paying attention.
- Spend time with siblings, including them if appropriate and possible.

Distraction and diversionary play and post-procedural play often takes place around or after specialised play preparation sessions. HPSs use a varied approach to supporting children throughout their hospital stay.

Specialised play – specific patient referrals

HPSs sometimes work with children and young people individually via a patient referral system. The main reasons why they would be referred for this additional support and interventions include anxiety about their hospital visit or diagnosis, fear of both the known and unknown elements of their treatment, distress due to a previous bad experience or because they are described as being 'non-compliant' by others within the MDT. Some children will have specific additional needs that mean they need more support during a hospital visit or admission. These additional needs include learning disabilities, a mental health condition, sensory issues, ADHD and autism.

Some hospitals have an established system in place for referrals, meaning that once a referral is received, a HPS is allocated to assist individual children. They liaise with the referrer, parent or carer and any other relevant health professional in relation to the needs of that child. The HPS then assesses whether any specialised play including preparation, distraction, desensitisation or general support would be appropriate on the day of the child or young person's appointment or admission, or whether they require a specialised preparation visit prior to admission. This could be a virtual preparation appointment if that is most suited to the needs of the child.

For some families, the HPS can send out information, social stories, photographs of the hospital and health professionals, links to useful apps, reward charts and other relevant resources to help alleviate any stress, anxiety and assist with communication about and preparation for hospital.

Since there is no agreed way of organising play services in the UK, referral systems vary between NHS trusts. However, evidence suggests that children who attend pre-admission days settle more quickly into their surroundings and are more relaxed and happy than those who did not (Keeton, 1999). The 2003 National Service Framework for Children also made clear recommendations that where admission to hospital is planned, children should be prepared through pre-admission play and information and that a visit to the ward should always be offered (Department of Health, 2003).

Conclusion

HPSs assist many children and young people including those who have a variety of complex needs, anxieties, fears and phobias and learning disabilities. Through their training and skills acquired through experience, HPSs use various techniques and strategies – described in this chapter under the umbrella term of 'specialised play' – to help children to master and cope with the stress of a hospital visit or admission. Specialised play has many benefits, and aims to meet the individual needs of children and young people in the hospital setting. By providing various forms of specialised therapeutic play and using clear, age-appropriate and developmentally appropriate communication, the work of the HPS has a positive impact on the health, well-being and recovery of children. Whether the child is a patient in outpatients, the Emergency Department, radiology, on a ward, in a spontaneous clinic visit or via a patient referral system, it is acknowledged that specialised play assists the process of being cared for in hospital and creates better outcomes for the children, young people and their families

References

Adams, J., Gill, S. & McDonald, M. (1991) Reducing Fears in Hospital. *Nursing Times* 87 (1), pp. 62–64

Bielby, E. (1984) A Childish Concept. *Nursing Mirror* 159 (18), pp. 26–28

Carson, D., Gravley, J. & Council, J. (1992) Children's Prehospitalization Conceptions of Illness, Cognitive Development and Personal Adjustment. *Children's Health Care* 21 (2), pp. 103–110

Department of Health (2003) *Getting the Right Start: National Service Framework for Children: Standard for Hospital Services.* London: Department of Health

Eiser, C. (1990) *Chronic Childhood Disease: An Introduction to Psychological Theory and Research.* Cambridge: Cambridge University Press

Fairclough, S. & Bennett, V. (2021) Play for Children and Young People in Hospital and Healthcare Settings, In: Glasper, E., Richardson, J. & Randall, D. (Eds) *A Textbook of Children and Young People's Nursing*, 3rd ed. London: Elsevier

Gilman, C. & Frauman, A. (1987) Use of Play with the Child and Chronic Illness. *American Nephrology Nurses' Association Journal* 14 (4), pp. 259–261

Glasper, E. & Thompson, M. (1993) Preparing Children for Hospital, In: Glasper E. & Tucker, A. (Eds) *Advances in Child Health Nursing.* London: Scutari Press

Heiney, S. (1991) Helping Children through Painful Procedures. *American Journal of Nursing* 91 (11), pp. 20–24

Hubbuck, C. (2009) *Play for Sick Children: Play Specialists in Hospital and Beyond.* London: Jessica Kingsley Publishers

Ivory, P. (1998) Taking the Scare out of Hospital Care for your Child. *Quest* 5 (3), pp. 1–6

Jolley, J. (2007) Separation and Psychological Trauma: A Paradox Examined. *Paediatric Nursing* 19 (3), pp. 22–25

Keeton, D. (1999) Pain, Nausea and Vomiting: A Day Surgery Audit. *Paediatric Nursing* 11 (5), pp. 28–32

Kool, R. & Lawver, T. (2010) Play Therapy: Considerations and Applications for the Practitioner. *Psychiatry (Edgmont)* 7 (10), pp. 19–24

Ministry of Health (1959) *The Welfare of Children in Hospital, Platt Report.* London: HMSO

Robertson, L. (1995) The Giving of Information Is the Key to Family Empowerment. *British Journal of Nursing* 4 (12), p. 692

Royal College of Paediatrics and Child Health (2019) *Facing the Future: Standards for Children in Emergency Care Settings.* [Online] Available from: <https://www.rcpch.ac.uk/resources/facing-future-standards-children-young-people-emergency-care-settings> [Accessed 18 July 2022]

Saile, H., Burgmeier, R. & Schmidt, I. (1988) A Meta-Analysis of Studies on Psychological Preparation of Children Facing Medical Procedures. *Psychology and Health* 2 (2), pp. 107–132

Vessey, J. & Mahon, M. (1990) Therapeutic Play and The Hospitalised Child. *Journal of Paediatric Nursing* 5 (5), pp. 328–333

Visintainer, M. & Wolfer, J. (1975) Psychological Preparation for Surgery Paediatric Patients: The Effects on Children's and Parents' Stress Responses and Adjustments. *Pediatrics* 56 (2), pp. 187–192

Walker, J. (2006) *Play for Health: Delivering and Auditing Quality in Hospital Play Services.* London: National Association of Hospital Play Specialists

While, A. (1994) Day Case Surgery. *Maternal Child Health* 19 (6), p. 1846

Whitebread, D. (2012) *The Importance of Play: A Report on the Value of Children's Play with a Series of Policy Recommendations.* Brussels: Toy Industries of Europe

12

THE ANGRY PLAY SPECIALIST

Cath Hubbuck – Senior Health Play Specialist

She was six years old. I didn't know her until I was asked to see her.

They wanted to trial a new treatment. They hoped it would improve her symptoms.

She was anxious. She had struggled at previous appointments.

The team were concerned – "Let's get Play involved".

So, I accepted the referral.

She was avoidant in the waiting room. Not charmed by me or my colouring or 'Connect Four' or my pop-beads. I had seen this before. Children can be avoidant when they are unsure of what is about to happen. It is – to some extent – a sign of healthy attachments and development. So I wasn't fazed. We were both checking each other out.

I popped briefly to the playroom. Then I heard her. The shrill wail of a child, scared and distressed, and in the background, the swell of multiple adult voices instructing her – both noises beating against each other.

In my two-minute absence she had been called, ushered into a four-bedded bay and asked to get on the bed. She was scared – terrified, even. Screaming and sobbing all at once, talking to her father in a language I didn't understand. She had hidden herself under the bed.

I dropped down to my knees – I know to get down really low for this – and over the noise still tried to use a gentle tone. "What's wrong?" I asked, directing my question to her, but hoping the father would translate. "She does not want anyone to hold her. She does not want to be held down", he replied for her.

"Will you let me help you?" I asked.

Slowly, with coaxing and the promise of play, she stopped hiding.

DOI: 10.4324/9781003255444-15

The completion of her treatment took over three hours. It was a complicated procedure.

Having managed to gain her trust, and invited her to sit on the bed, and assisted her nurse in obtaining her baseline observations, there was topical anaesthetic cream and a sticky dressing to apply to each leg. These both had to be removed after half an hour. Then the procedure itself involved the insertion of a fine needle into each thigh. Then an infusion that needed to run through for 90 minutes. Then there was the removal of more adhesive dressings and finally the needles.

It was relentless for her. I think it was relentless for all of us. Each part held particular difficulties. Each part required the rebuilding and strengthening of trust, the encouragement to sit still, the need to endure discomfort, the courage to face very real fears and all the way through, the effort to communicate backwards and forwards through her father. Gradually the reasons for her fearfulness were understood. Gradually reassurance was given that – if we worked together – we would not resort to her deeply felt and overwhelming fear of being held against her will.

Through her father, I learned that she had faced many hospital appointments, procedures and admissions. However, her fear had been established after being held down for the placement of a naso-gastric tube when she was four years old. She said, as we played during her infusion, "They just all came in and they held me and I could not move. I felt like I might not be alive".

Such honesty. Such a vivid recollection. I could understand the root of her terror.

And yet, we managed it – all of it.

I praised her for her bravery. I could see she was exhausted, but we parted with a happy high-five.

I left work grateful for the walk home that day. The encounter with this little girl troubled me. It had been an extraordinary day for her, I reflected, but my own days frequently hold complex, lengthy and sometimes distressing experiences like this. I often leave work still thinking deeply and processing the things I have encountered in my working day.

As I walked, I realised I felt angry – really angry.

Sometimes I really am an angry play specialist.

I love my job. I really do. But when I recall that day – and all the days like it – anger still swells inside me. Of course, I rarely express that anger – at least, not at work. Can you imagine that? The jolly, friendly, development-promoting, toy-providing, noise-making, glitter-sprinkling, messy play-enjoying, endlessly patient play specialist – your multidisciplinary team (MDT) 'phone-a-friend'. And, when all is said and done, everyone seems to comment on what a great and happy job it must be. Surely, there is no room for anger? And yet … still those feelings arise.

I have been a health play specialist (HPS) for more than 20 years and I think I have been more angry recently than ever before. During that time, I have tried to nurture a more reflective and deductive approach to considering the impact of my work. So, maybe I have been more angry recently – or maybe I am just becoming more aware of feeling angry and more curious about why. Maybe I have become more open to trying to understand it in context and to address it.

There is a saying, a variation on a quote originally attributed to C.S. Lewis:

"I sat with my anger long enough for it to tell me its real name was sadness".

Reframed this way, there can be curiosity about whether there are other things at play, aside from simply grumpiness or outrage. We can wonder about the aspects of the HPS's work that might be the cause of 'sadness' – or if not 'sadness' then perhaps other deep or more complex feelings of a similar quality – frustration, distress or overwhelm, for example? As practitioners who recognise the value of reflection (HPSET, 2019), it is important and useful to observe and acknowledge the potential for feelings to arrive in us during the challenges brought by our work. However, regular clinical supervision is rarely available to HPSs working within the National Health Service (NHS) and – as a result – it is possible for many practitioners that difficult or uncomfortable feelings arising from practice are not given space to be recognised or processed. That is part of what makes the work of HPSs so challenging as much as it is also enjoyable and rewarding.

Given this, when I reflect upon feeling angry in the course of my work with sick children – when I ask myself the question "What is really happening here?" – I am left more aware of the things that consistently make the work of being a HPS a tough call. None of these are unique or particular to the scenario I have shared and yet all of them are things that, I believe, contributed to my reactions that day and potentially those reactions of many other colleagues to the work that is undertaken by HPSs every day.

The expectations placed on HPSs

The work of the HPS has changed considerably in the years since the inception of the role in the UK. Training has been developed and the HPS has been accepted within NHS MDTs. With this the breadth, depth and scope of the HPS's practice has increased (Kennedy, 2010; Tonkin, 2014), with individual practitioners becoming deeply knowledgeable in particular clinical specialities (Brindle, 2006; Gill, 2013). While positive, the greater the demands placed on HPSs as practitioners inevitably adds to the potential for a higher emotional and psychological burden on them both professionally and personally.

HPSs are skilled in responding practically to the needs of children and families in highly distressing circumstances. They assist with invasive medical procedures and do so repeatedly, frequently adjusting and tempering their approach to take into account the requirements of the clinical setting, the short and longer-term implications of each procedure and the specific needs of every child. Some colleagues refer to this as 'magic'. "Let's get play involved", they say, calling on HPSs to "work their magic" on distressed patients. But it is not magic. It is a set of skills, knowledge and experience that informs good practice.

Within their practice, often with very short notice and very little time or physical space, HPSs are asked to help by colleagues who have an expectation that 'a little bit of playing' will make everything 'nice' or at least bearable for the child, who may be distressed or already traumatised. Children in hospital have often experienced a complex, multi-layered mixture of traumatic events (GOSH, 2020). They may have faced and may continue to face traumatic experience after traumatic experience, at different times, in different healthcare settings and their behavioural responses may be different every time. Whenever they attend the hospital, there is another invasive procedure, or examination, or consultation to be completed.

As I worked with my patient, I was not only responsible for facilitating her coping in the face of a new challenging and invasive medical procedure but also for doing so in the context of previous medical experiences that had been terrifying for her. Controversial though it may be to say it, I am often required to deal with the 'mishandling' of children by other people. This may be care which is well intentioned – life-saving even – but which nonetheless leads to children facing each subsequent procedure in a terrified state – a traumatised state. We do not name trauma enough and I believe we should do so more often. By not naming it, we also fail to acknowledge what challenges there are in working with individuals – adults or children – struggling with the effects of trauma.

Under such circumstances, it is a testament to the skill, patience and intuition of HPSs when things go well. However, in spite of this, the pressure on and expectations of HPSs is often unrealistic and unreasonable. At all times the HPSs must acknowledge each child's previous experiences of overwhelming trauma, their current anxious anticipation of pain *and* get them successfully through another procedure. That is a tough call.

The cost of compassion for the experiences of children and their families

Children with significant illness or injury endure extraordinary things within the hospital setting. Repeated invasive procedures, even if ultimately for good reasons, are an assault on the body. Scans, intra-venous infusions, the insertion of lines, the insertion of rods, the removal of organs, hair-loss, immobility, anticipatory anxiety, pain, disruptions to sleep, nutrition and recreation as well as the separation from home and school are variously faced. Generally speaking, children cope stoically – some days are better than others, some things more bearable than others. And as part of the healthcare team, we bear witness to it all – the good, the bad and the downright ugly. These are things that happen behind closed hospital doors. Confidentiality is rightly maintained for all our patients, but often the experiences of sick children have to be seen to be believed.

Invasive medical procedures are still one of the more commonly overlooked sources of children's trauma (Levine and Klein, 2007). They are not the experiences of your average six yearold, and, as such, children in hospital experience things that are beyond the scope of their usual everyday lives before they became ill or injured. It is within the HPS's role to rapidly help them learn to understand and to cope with things well beyond the level of their development. HPSs are there for them throughout, with paint and dolls and slime and cheeriness and companionship to help them make-meaning and help them keep-on keeping-on, day after day after day. That is a tough call.

What drives this work? I believe it is compassion – defined as being "a strong feeling of sympathy or sadness for the suffering ... of others and a wish to help them" (Cambridge Dictionary 2020). The drive in HPSs to respond to children with compassion is what makes the work so powerful and often so effective. It is also what can make it so emotionally costly. Furthermore, when the trauma experienced by children in hospitals is properly acknowledged, so too comes an acknowledgement that all those working closely with them are at risk of compassion stress and vicarious trauma.

Compassion stress – the stress 'connected with exposure to a person who is suffering' (Figley, 1998, p. 21) – is widely acknowledged as a risk for those working within caring professions (Quitangon, 2019). Vicarious trauma is more specifically acknowledged as a 'psychological hazard' faced by those in health-care settings, especially when their exposure to distressing or traumatic circumstances is repeated – as it undoubtedly is in the case of many HPSs. The British Medical Association (2022) has stated that anyone who engages empathetically with people facing traumatic incidents can be affected by vicarious trauma and that this can lead to a change in the outlook and self-perception of practitioners. Warning signs of this include lingering feelings of anger, rage and sadness about the patient's situation. Given my own emotional response to my encounter with my young patient, this is an interesting point and worthy of note for HPSs as practitioners. Unchecked or unacknowledged, compassion stress and vicarious trauma can progress to 'compassion fatigue' – broadly known as 'burnout'.

So what now?

Much of the work of the HPS – and even the job title itself – suggests that we are predominantly providers of play. Beyond this however, the baseline, foundational aspects of the work are actually concerned with reducing and responding to children's distress and trauma. In acknowledging this, it is clear that for all the joy that is found in play, the HPS's job is stressful. It is a role which alongside all its enrichment and enjoyment – mutually experienced between children and practitioners – is challenging and sometimes difficult. It is also one where, as practitioners, HPSs regularly encounter acute suffering, profound sadness and extreme distress in others, and to a greater or lesser extent, experience these emotions for themselves too. It is important to acknowledge that the nature of the HPSs work, the placement of their role within the MDT and the physical place they often undertake during invasive procedures puts them at an increased, acute and ongoing risk of emotional and psychological difficulties caused by vicarious trauma.

A difficulty for play staff in hospitals is that the stress they experience is in danger of going unacknowledged by others on the MDT. This is largely because – as non-clinical practitioners – we play, and play is so often considered to be joyful, light-hearted and fun. Our role encompasses all of these things and more but, because we play within the clinical environment of the hospital, that work brings with it challenges not encountered in other spaces where play is provided. The HPS must hold carefully the tension between acknowledging children's distress and extending compassionate support, while assisting during upsetting invasive procedures. To consistently respond to a child's needs with playfulness and with empathy to their trauma is a challenge, the reality of which cannot be adequately taught or prepared for in our training. This work can be overwhelming. This work can affect you in ways you were not expecting. This work can be enormously rewarding – guiding and supporting children through challenging circumstances – but it requires the development of an awareness of what is happening in terms of emotional and psychological well-being. That is a tough call.

Sometimes I really am an angry play specialist – but I know those feelings arise because sometimes the work I do is hard and unrelenting; and because it is difficult to witness children suffering; and because sometimes I feel powerless to change the experiences of those children; or because the expectations placed on me to help children are too high.

My anger can be uncomfortable, but it is important to notice what it is really telling me.

Ultimately, I am a human being. And that alone is quite a tough call.

References

Brindle, L. (2006) 'The case for play in a neonatal intensive care unit – The work of a hospital play specialist' in *Journal of Neonatal Nursing* Vol 12 (issue 1), pp. 14–19

British Medical Association (2022) Vicarious trauma: Signs and strategies for coping. [Online] Available from: <https://www.bma.org.uk/advice-and-support/your-wellbeing/vicarious-trauma/vicarious-trauma-signs-and-strategies-for-coping> [Accessed 4 February 2022]

Cambridge Dictionary (2020) *Cambridge Advanced Learner's Dictionary & Thesaurus.* [Online] Available from: <https://dictionary.cambridge.org/dictionary/english/compassion> [Accessed 14 February 2022]

Figley, C. (1998) Burnout as Systemic Traumatic Stress: A Model for Helping Traumatized Family Members. pp. 15–28. In: Figley, C. (ed.) *Burnout in Families: The Systemic Costs of Caring.* Boca Raton, FL: CRC Press LLC

Gill, C. (2013) 'Helping children cope with renal disease: The role of the play specialist' in *Journal of Renal Nursing* Vol 2 (issue 5). [Online] Available from: <https://www.magonlinelibrary.com/doi/abs/10.12968/jorn.2010.2.5.78490> [Accessed 7 February 2022]

GOSH (2020) *Supporting Children and Young People after a Traumatic Hospital Admission.* Great Ormond Street Hospital for Children. [Online] Available from: <https://www.gosh.nhs.uk/conditions-and-treatments/procedures-and-treatments/supporting-children-and-young-people-after-traumatic-hospital-admission/> [Accessed 17 February 2022]

Hospital Play Specialist Education Trust (HPSET) (2019) *Standards of Proficiency and Professional Standards.* [Online] Available from: <https://hpset.org.uk/HPSET_ps.pdf> [Accessed 15 February 2022]

Kennedy, I. (2010) *Getting It Right for Children and Young People: Overcoming Cultural Barriers in the NHS so as to Meet their Needs.* London: Department of Health

Levine P. & Klein, M. (2007) *Trauma through a Child's Eyes.* Berkeley CA: North Atlantic Books

Quitangon, G. (2019) 'Vicarious trauma in clinicians: Fostering resilience and preventing burnout' in *Psychiatric Times* Vol 36 (issue 7). [Online] Available from: <https://www.psychiatrictimes.com/view/vicarious-trauma-clinicians-fostering-resilience-and-preventing-burnout> [Accessed 15 February 2022]

Tonkin, A. (2014) *The Provision of Play in Health Service Delivery: A Literature Review.* London: NAHPS

PART III

Specific case studies

13

SUPPORT FOR CHILDREN AND YOUNG PEOPLE UNDERGOING RADIOTHERAPY TREATMENT

Lobke Marsden – Health Play Specialist

While a cancer diagnosis is rare in children and young people, there have been around 75,000 young people diagnosed with cancer over the last 20 years, which is approximately 3,755 per year (Irvine, 2021). This translates to around 33,000 cases diagnosed in children (0–14 year olds), an average of 1,645 cases per year, and 42,000 cases for teenage and young adults (15–24 year olds), which is roughly 2,110 per year. In Leeds we have an average of around 50–70 patients a year, being referred to us with a cancer diagnosis, for radiotherapy treatment.

What is radiotherapy?

Radiotherapy is a treatment where radiation is used to treat and kill cancer cells (NHS, 2020). Over 50% of people with cancer need radiotherapy as part of their treatment plan. Radiotherapy can be used to eliminate cancer cells, reduce the chance of them returning, or it can be used to relieve symptoms caused by cancer. This treatment can be given before, during and after other cancer treatments such as chemotherapy, surgery, immunotherapy and endocrine therapy, or it can be given as a sole treatment.

Radiotherapy aims to destroy the cancer cells in the area that is being treated. Radiation damages the DNA inside cancer cells causing them to stop growing, become unable to repair, and thus, stop multiplying (Cancer Research UK, 2020). The cancerous cells are not able to recover from the damage caused by the radiation, and that results in a reduction or elimination of the cancer cells. Unfortunately, radiation also affects healthy cells, and it is this that can cause side effects. However, healthy non-cancerous cells are better able to recover from exposure to radiation (Radiotherapy UK, 2022).

Most of our patients require some kind of device that helps them lie completely still for their radiotherapy treatment. The kind of device needed will

DOI: 10.4324/9781003255444-17

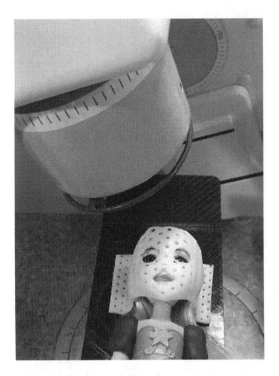

FIGURE 13.1 Doll on a machine with toy mask.

depend on the part of the patient's body that needs treating. For example, a lot of our patients have a brain tumour, so children and young people will need to wear a radiotherapy mask whilst being treated. This mask is clipped to the bed, which means the patient cannot move, allowing for treatment precision (Figure 13.1).

On average patients tend to have six weeks of radiotherapy treatment, Monday to Fridays, with the weekends off, but this depends entirely on their diagnosis and treatment plan.

The role of the health play specialist in radiotherapy

Undergoing radiotherapy treatment can be a daunting and challenging experience regardless of the age of the patient. My main role as a play specialist is to support patients through these challenges and help to make their radiotherapy treatment experience the best it can be while trying to reduce the risk of trauma. This would not be possible without a level of trust. Trust is the basis of every meaningful relationship, and it is needed for a child/young person (YP) to feel in control, during a time when this is not always possible. In my opinion trust and control are the two most important elements that contribute to the possibility of a child successfully managing their radiotherapy treatment (Figure 13.2).

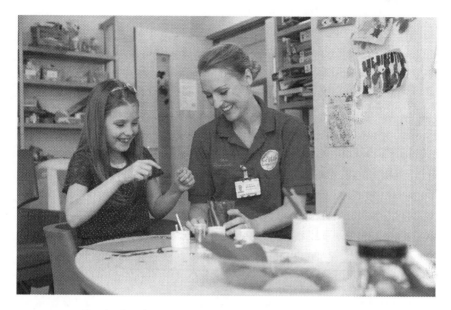

FIGURE 13.2 Fun in the play room.

When a patient is referred to our department, and if time allows, I meet the patient to find out their likes/dislikes without even a mention of radiotherapy. I try to gain their trust and establish a connection through their interests. Christmas time, a few years ago we had a little girl, aged 6, coming over for an introductory chat with the doctor. I was told by the team that she would need a radiotherapy mask for her treatment and that would likely be very challenging for her as she was very scared of any hospital procedures, due to traumatic experiences in the past at another hospital.

The day I met her she was very scared and hardly made eye contact with me when I introduced myself. She chose to sit close to her parents and did not want to join me at the art and craft table. After keeping my distance for a little while, I asked her if it was okay for me to sit next to her, to which she quietly said yes. I moved a few crafts to the table where she was sitting and without saying anything I started to create something from the art materials. She started to show some interest in what I was doing and passed me the glue when needed without me even asking her. After a little while she started to pick up materials for herself and before long we were both crafting. The atmosphere had changed, and I noticed she felt comfortable and safe in my company – even when her parents briefly left the room to speak to the doctor.

I had already been told by her parents that Santa would be bringing her a very special present; a Reborn Doll she had asked for. As it happened my little girl had also asked for a Reborn Doll. Before she left the department, I told her of the doll my little girl was hoping to get for Christmas. In that moment she forgot she did not want to talk to me and shouted out: "So did I!" I asked if she wanted to see a picture of the doll my daughter had her eye on, which she did. She then instructed her mum to show me a picture of her much-wanted doll on her phone. I asked the girl if she would come back to show me her doll if Santa did bring it, which she nodded her head in response. She left the department a completely different girl compared to when she arrived. We connected and this created an opening for the start of treatment preparation in the weeks that followed.

When this little girl returned a week later, proudly showing me the doll Santa gave her, we spent a day playing and crafting together – strengthening the trust between us. She returned again after this session, only then did I slowly introduce radiotherapy and the idea of having a mask made for the treatment. To break this down, a mask was first made on her hand so she could get used to the sensation of the warm material and later she helped make a mask on her dad to familiarise herself with the process. Only then she felt ready to have one made for herself. She felt in control throughout, and we went at her pace. The outcome would have likely been very different had she been rushed into having a radiotherapy mask made without the previous sessions offered beforehand, and this little girl then went on to have her treatment without the need of a general anaesthetic.

Something that we do for all of our patients, up to the age of 25, is to have their radiotherapy mask painted in a design of their choice (Figure 13.3).

The first mask we painted was in 2016 for a four-year-old patient who asked for a Spiderman radiotherapy mask. I will never forget his excitement over having his

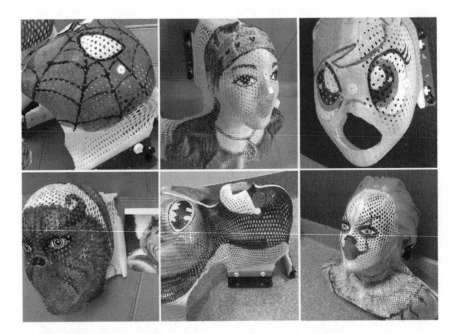

FIGURE 13.3 Six little masks.

mask made, knowing it would soon become his Spiderman mask. He even came dressed as Spiderman to his mould room appointment and did so for most of his radiotherapy treatments afterwards. It was the first time I had actually seen a child get excited over having their radiotherapy mask made. It was then that I realised this was so much more than a little bit of paint.

Although some children and YP quite enjoy the feeling of having a radiotherapy mask made (some compare it to having a facial due to the warm sensation of the warm orfit material) – for most of our patients having a mask made can be a little challenging. The main challenges can be having their eyes covered, feeling claustrophobic by having their face covered or not liking the warmth of the mask – especially if this concerns a child/YP who is particularly sensitive to sensory sensations. I will always tell the patient they are in control, and they only have to lift their hand if they would like the mask to be taken off straight away. As the patient is encouraged not to talk whilst having their mask made (to not alter the shape of the mask) we communicate by responding with thumbs up to let us know they are happy for us to continue. I talk to the child/YP throughout, telling them what is happening and what stage we are at or how much longer it is likely to take.

Some patients who are very anxious benefit from guided imagery. We discuss this beforehand, and they choose a happy memory. When they are calm and relaxed, I ask them to describe this to me in great detail – smells, sights any small little thing to really take them back to that moment. A six-year-old boy who was very anxious about having his mask made told me about his trip to Disneyland. He described the parade to me and told me all the characters that were at the front and the ones that followed. During his mask making session he asked for Disney music to be played very softly in the background while I held his hand and in a calm voice spoke to him about all the wonderful things he had told me about this parade in Disneyland. You could see him relax by the rise and fall of his chest slowing down. His hand grip loosened, and before he knew it his mask had been made.

With our very young patients there is often an element of role play involved where they take on traits of the character they chose to have painted on their masks. We have been told that some feel "brave" like the superhero on their mask whilst wearing it for treatment. Another young girl who had lost all her hair due to chemotherapy, asked me to paint the hair she lost on her mask as she felt more confident with her hair. She was very specific describing how she wanted this to look and helped me mix the right colour, right down to highlights to exactly match the hair she had lost and missed having.

By allowing patients to choose the design of their radiotherapy mask we can give them back some control. We have been told by a young adult patient that having "a say", even over something as simple as a design, meant a great deal to him. He told us how so far, he had had no say in his treatment, or where he was having this, how long for, etc., but during this time he did. Because of this personalisation he said his mask no longer felt like a cold clinical device, but it felt like HIS. Because of this personalisation he grew attached to it. Even now, years after treatment, he still has it proudly displayed on a shelf in his bedroom and he tells us it reminds him of what he has gone through and how far he has come.

As well as offering mask painting, we offer patients young and old the use of "magic string" during treatment. Magic string is a simple long multicoloured piece of string that becomes magical the moment a patient begins their treatment simply by still feeling connected to their loved one holding the other side. The patient lies on the bed holding on to the string with their chosen person holding the other end, from a different room. Because of the radiation, patients must be on their own in the treatment room during their radiotherapy. This can be quite tricky, especially if parents have been able to sit with their children during previous scans. Separation anxiety can be a real challenge – mainly at their first treatment when the child will be a little anxious and apprehensive, wondering what to expect. The magic string can really help as the child/YP no longer feels left on their own and feels reassured their loved one is right on the other side of the string. They can give it a little reassuring tug to let them know they are still there and even though they are in the treatment room by themselves – they are not alone. A five-year-old boy told us that to him it felt like still holding hands with his mummy (Figure 13.4).

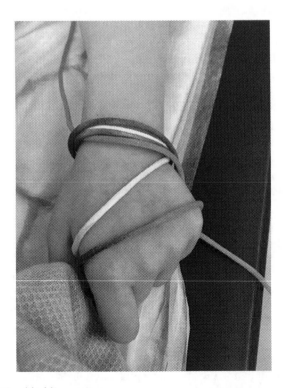

FIGURE 13.4 Hand holding string.

Something as simple and cheap as string has prevented many general anaesthetics in the past for children who struggle with separation anxiety. We have found it to be equally comforting to parents, as well as their children, as it must be very difficult to leave your child on their own during treatment.

I have recently received a thank you card from a patient's mother. She wrote:

> You played a significant part in helping L cope and feel at ease, earning his trust through calming and creative play. We think you went above and beyond to help L feel secure.

Those words really touched me and made me realise that "play" is not just play. It is so much more. It allows us to connect, validate, offer security, expression and a safe way to help patients through what could have been a traumatic hospital experience. A little boy once called our hospital the play hospital, where he just happened to have some treatment in between play sessions. It doesn't get much more rewarding than that.

References

Cancer Research UK (2020) *What is radiotherapy?* [Online] Available from: <https://www.cancerresearchuk.org/about-cancer/cancer-in-general/treatment/radiotherapy/about> [Accessed 18 May 2020]

Irvine, L. (2021) *Cancer in children and young people – what do the statistics tell us?* [Online] https://ukhsa.blog.gov.uk/2021/03/15/cancer-in-children-and-young-people-what-do-the-statistics-tell-us/ [Accessed 22 June 2022]

NHS (2020) *Radiotherapy.* [Online] Available from: <https://www.nhs.uk/conditions/radiotherapy/> [Accessed 18 May 2022]

Radiotherapy UK (2022) *What is radiotherapy?* [Online] Available from: <https://radiotherapy.org.uk> [Accessed 18 May 2022]

14

WORKING WITH CHILDREN AND YOUNG PEOPLE WITH AUTISM IN THE HEALTH CARE SETTING

Nicola Voos – Registered and Qualified Health Play Specialist and FE Teacher

Susan Fairclough – Therapeutic and Specialised Play Service Manager, Youth Service Manager and Events Lead

Autism is something we are constantly learning about. This chapter focuses on the vital role of the health play specialist (HPS) in assisting children, young people and adults who have learning disabilities or are on the autistic spectrum. We discuss what it is like for these people coming into hospital for examinations, procedures, treatments, and surgery. We offer a snapshot of the HPS role through a real case scenario which is provided alongside quotes from other authors and specialists within this field. We also highlight the relevant links to the Health Play Specialist Education Trust which is the organisation and governing body that all HPSs should be registered with.

Before discussing the health play specialist's (HPS's) role let's look at what autism is. Autism Spectrum Disorder (ASD) is a relatively common neurodevelopmental condition. The definition of autism is based on the presence of impairments in social communication, social interaction and restricted, repetitive patterns of behaviours interests or activities. These impairments vary greatly in severity and whilst often noticeable during childhood can go undetected until later in life (NINDS 2022).

The term 'autistic' was first used in 1908 by Dr Eugen Bleuler. Autism comes from the Greek word 'auto' meaning self. Leo Kanner, a psychiatrist, went on to study young men that had a need for sameness or a resistance to unexpected change (Kanner 1943). Hans Asperger (1944) describes children with similar clinical features to Kanner's young people. However, Asperger's descriptions were different in the areas of communication, motor and fine skills and learning styles. Wing and Gould (1979) provided the next major influential additions to research literature and clinical practice when they published the 'triad of impairments' which grouped the features of autism, social interaction, communication,

DOI: 10.4324/9781003255444-18

and imagination and led to the understanding of difficulties with theory of mind. This led to the publication of the Autistic Spectrum (Wing 1996).

> Autism is a lifelong developmental disability which affects how people communicate and interact with the world. One in 100 people are on the autism spectrum and there are around 700,000 autistic adults and children in the UK
>
> *National Autistic Society (2022)*

As the National Autistic Society shows, autism is common and is now recognised as a condition that requires society to change the way it provides communication and recognise the need to make services autism friendly. Autism has a large spectrum, some children, young people, and adults can function within their normal day to day life but struggle with change and social interaction, yet others may also have a learning disability that impacts their ability to develop skills such as verbal communication and understanding the world around them.

In the UK healthcare is a service that should be accessible to all. This means healthcare providers have a legal obligation to ensure that all professionals within their organisation receive training relating to the Equality Act 2010 and the Care Act 2014, these legislations along with many more are then used to provide policies, procedures, and guidelines for staff who have direct contact with service users. All healthcare professionals are required to complete annual training on equality, diversity, safeguarding, moving and handling, etc. This has been the case for many years meaning that all health professionals have a duty to make reasonable adjustments as part of their practice to meet the needs of service users with a disability (Disability Discrimination Act 1995).

> On Thursday 28th April, the Oliver McGowan Mandatory Training in Learning Disability and Autism passed into law as part of the Health and Care Act 2022, following strong support by the government to legislate for mandatory training across the health and care sectors.
>
> *Mencap (2022)*

This followed the preventable death of Oliver McGowan after the professionals ignored Oliver and his parents, and gave him a medication that had previously had a negative effect on him. Oliver was 18 years old and had mild learning difficulties and autism. This case highlighted the failings of health professionals as they felt they had the authority to bypass Oliver's rights even though he had mental capacity and his next of kin disagreed with their decision. "People with a learning disability are more likely to die avoidably and die younger than the general population" (Mencap 2022). This law should ensure that vital training in the health and social care sector means people with a learning disability and people with autism get the health and care support they need.

Although organisations have a legal obligation to ensure their services are accessible to all and that professionals have the appropriate training, individuals with autism may still need extra assistance to be able to cope with the healthcare environment.

> Children and young people with Autistic Spectrum Disorder (ASD) can react to hospital admission in different ways and having access to a staff member with appropriate training and experience can reduce distress and improve the patient and staff experience.
>
> *Pratt et al. (2012)*

Staff members may be working in the role of a learning disability nurse, Autism Specialist or a HPS; whatever their title they all share the same goal, i.e. to provide a service that is person-centred and meets an individual's holistic and healthcare needs.

While all paediatric health professionals can use play in their care of the child or young person, the HPS holds the responsibility for ensuring the essential functions of play are built into the fabric of the child's or young person's journey through the hospital experience (Walker 2006). This is highlighted in developmental, therapeutic, and specialised play intervention. HPSs, unlike any other staff, have as their major responsibility the social and emotional welfare of the child, young person, and family (Hogg 1990).

For those children and young people, it may be their first visit to hospital, or they may be a regular patient. All children and young people's experiences are different, and their personalities, feelings, emotions, and needs are all unique. It is therefore important to listen to each child and young person and their family to assess their individual needs.

The role of the HPS has evolved over the years and is vital in meeting children and young people's needs in all areas of healthcare. More and more services are recognising this role, including hospices, care in the community and private sector provision. HPSs offer developmental, therapeutic, and specialised play for children and young people in the hospital/healthcare setting. They liaise closely with the patient, their family, and many health professionals who are all working in collaboration to provide the best possible holistic care and a positive experience for the patient and family.

HPSs help patients prepare for hospital or the healthcare environment via patient referrals, pre-admission work, in-patient work, psychological and specialised preparation for treatments, procedures and surgery, whilst also offering distraction, diversional or participation therapies during procedures and post procedural play and intervention.

HPSs undertake individual patient referrals besides undertaking the ward/department patient activity. They can assist children and young people by preparing them for the hospital setting, treatment, procedures, and surgery where a trusting therapeutic relationship is deepened through play (Kool and Lawver 2010).

Some children/young people who attend hospital have additional needs, learning disabilities, communication difficulties or they are on the autistic spectrum and require be-spoke care packages and intervention. The process that takes place to be able to make these bespoke packages often starts with contacting the family prior to their child or young person's healthcare visit. The National Autistic Society have developed a 'hospital passport' which can be downloaded from their website and completed by the individual with autism and/or someone who is familiar to them. This could be a family member, a friend, or a professional. However, some organisations take it one step further and follow processes such as those in Figure 14.1 (see next page).

This process is something that may need repeating a number of times for individuals who access the services on an ad-hoc or regular basis, the reason this process is repeated is to continue in providing person-centred care. One of the reasons for this is that the service users' interests, requirements or fears may change over time, so what works for one visit or admission may not work the next time, and adequate planning needs to allow for this. It is also a good practice to reflect on the individual's experience after they have attended the healthcare setting, a good way to do this is to allow families to complete evaluation forms or contact the family after the visit/admission to discuss their experience. This can include areas for improvement and the positive effects of careful planning and working in partnership with families and other professionals.

The Healthcare Play Specialist Education Trust (HPSET)

HPSET is the governing body for HPSs. All HPSs must continue with professional development not only in the form of annual mandatory training outlined above but also within the context of their own role. They must re-register annually. They are required to maintain a record of their professional development and submit a portfolio, profile of evidence to support this, every three years. They also must work within the HPSET Code of Professional Conduct (2013) and the HPSET Professional Standards (2019). Items of relevance to working with individuals on the autistic spectrum include:

Code of Professional Conduct for Registered Practitioners and Students

5.2 To support standards of practice you must take every opportunity to maintain and improve professional knowledge and competence.

5.5 Listen to service users, their families, and carers and take account of their needs and wishes.

6.4 At all times safeguard the well-being and interests of children, young people, and their families and carers, taking into consideration the physical, psychological, and social effect of the environment and situation.

HPSET (2013)

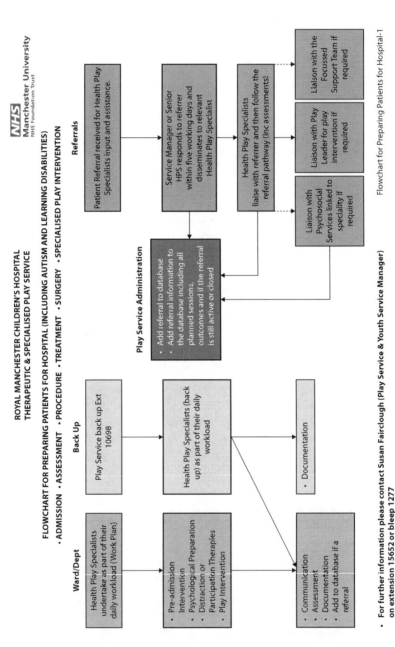

FIGURE 14.1 Manchester University NHS Foundation Trust – Royal Manchester Children's Hospital, Therapeutic and Specialised Play Service – flowchart for preparing patients for hospital (including autistic and learning disabilities).

Health Play Specialist Standards of Proficiency and Professional Standards

2.8 To embed the 6C's of value-based care into daily practice.

4.1 Be able to assess a professional situation, to determine the nature and severity of a problem, and to act within your professional scope of practice at all times.

4.5 To facilitate choice and control through patient-centred care, using play-based techniques that support positive outcomes.

4.5a Be able to work in partnership with other professionals to ensure that clinical procedures are planned and managed, enabling a consistent and compassionate approach by the team.

8.5 Understand the need to assist the communication of service users, such as an appropriate interpreter, assistive technology, and other support systems.

14.6 Be able to develop or modify play activities for service users, to build on their abilities and enhance their experience.

HPSET (2019)

The following section consists of events that occurred in preparation for and during a pre-admission appointment and on the day of surgery. All events are related to the same service user. The HPS ensured that the HPSET codes referred to above were adhered to at all times.

SCENARIO

Part 1 – A dentist from the dental hospital sent a written referral to the therapeutic and specialised play service via the online referral system. This was for a teenage girl who required a pre-admission appointment and then dental extractions under a general anaesthetic. The referral was sent to the play services because the girl has autism and severe learning difficulties.

Part 2 – A HPS contacted the mother to discuss the pre-admission and dental extraction admission and to carry out a person-centred assessment, during this time mum made the HPS aware that both herself and her husband were extremely concerned about the pre-admission appointment and the dental surgery. Mum stated that all dental examinations have previously taken place in the home whilst parents had to momentarily restrain their daughter as she would lash out due to fear. Mum also had concerns about entering the hospital and other people being around as this would cause distress to her daughter. The HPS reassured mum and explained that an alternative pathway could be arranged, which included reasonable adjustments in accessing the hospital, undergoing the pre-admission and on the day of surgery.

Part 3 – The HPS contacted the pre-admission team, the anaesthetic department, and the dental team to organise a combined appointment for the patient. Once all professionals had confirmed a date and time, the HPS contacted the security department to arrange the unlocking of a side fire exit that led straight into the dental clinic. The dental department had also agreed to a one-hour time slot where no other patients would be in the clinic. The HPS then contacted mum and informed her that a disabled car space would be reserved immediately outside the fire exit, where the family would be met by her and taken straight into the dental clinic.

Part 4 – The HPS devised a social story of the journey into hospital which included photographs of the areas and the people she would see. This included the HPS, pre-admission nurse, the dentist, and the anaesthetist she would see on the day of pre-admission. This was e-mailed to mum so that she could add to it, mum included their house, car, mum, dad and her daughter's favourite teddy and iPad.

Part 5 – The pre-admission appointment. The family arrived and parked in the reserved car space, the HPS met them at the car, and they all entered the dental waiting area, the only other person in this area was the dentist. Dad sat with his daughter (the patient), and they watched her favourite programme on the iPad, the patient showed me her favourite teddy, she was non-verbal, so dad talked to me on her behalf, and the patient used some basic Makaton signs. The dentist watched from afar and discussed the surgery with mum. The dentist then walked towards us; the HPS told the patient that this was her friend, and then did the Makaton sign for hello to the dentist, the patient then did the same. Dad was then encouraged to make his daughter laugh, he did this, and as she laughed, she tilted her head back and opened her mouth whilst laughing. As this was happening the dentist shone a torch into the patient's mouth and was able to look inside for a few seconds. Parents asked if they need to hold open their daughter's mouth for longer. The dentist informed them that she got a clear look at her teeth and could see at least four that needed removing at the back due to severe decay. Mum then went into a consultation room with a pre-admission nurse and dentist for approximately 20 minutes. Whilst this was happening the patient played on the football table with dad and the HPS. The anaesthetist was then bleeped by the pre-admission nurse and attended to go over the anaesthetic with mum. The HPS also attended this appointment, and a plan was discussed for the admission and the surgery. Part of this discussion was that mum would return on her own and the HPS would walk her through the route from entering the building, to her cubicle, to the operating theatre department and back out to the car. After this the family left the department through the fire exit.

NB. The hospital is now in the process of creating an accessible, planned separate and quiet entrance away from the busy entrance to accommodate patients who require this reasonable adjustment.

Part 6 – Mum attended to visit the areas her daughter would go, and the HPS walked her through two ways into the hospital and on to the ward. Mum chose the back door route which was the ambulance access to the neonatal department. Mum wanted to make her own social story so took lots of pictures of the route in, the ward corridor, a cubicle, the operating theatre waiting area, anaesthetic area, and the recovery area. She also took photographs of her daughter's favourite teddy on the hospital bed and a picture of a medicine syringe as well as the blood pressure machine, oximeter, and thermometer. The HPS then placed each of them onto the teddy whilst mum took photographs. The HPS gave mum an anaesthetic mask, a cannula with the needle removed, a bandage, and a syringe. Mum said the school nurse had agreed to weigh her daughter the day before admission and familiarise her with the blood pressure machine and oximeter at school.

Part 7 – (Dental Surgery). The HPS met the family at 08.00. The patient was placed in her wheelchair and taken down the back corridor and into a lift and then straight onto her ward and into her cubicle, at mum's request there was no bedding on the bed as she had brought her own, and no toys as again she brought her own. Whilst the family waited for the lift the HPS took the bedding and toys and went up the staircase and set up the cubicle, when the family entered the cubicle the patient unfastened her seatbelt, climbed out of her wheelchair and jumped on the bed, she then went over to the window and watched people walking past. The patient's weight (taken by the school nurse) was used to prescribe a pre-med. The patient allowed all observations to be done. Mum did her temperature as mum usually does it at home, so her daughter was familiar with the process. The anaesthetist then entered the room. All consent had been done during the pre-admission visit and parents where happy to proceed. The anaesthetist then drew up the pre-med and handed it to mum to give in a syringe. The patient took the pre-med and mum got her to lie on her bed and watch her iPad, so the HPS and anaesthetist waited at the door until the pre-med appeared to take effect. The patient fell asleep after 20 minutes. Mum and dad were allowed to attend the anaesthetic area. The HPS waited outside. After surgery it was agreed that the HPS would stay with the patient during the first stage of recovery and parents would be allowed to wait in the operating theatre waiting area. As soon as the patient started to come round the HPS went to get the parents. The patient recovered well and was able to have something to eat and drink, she played with her toys and watched her iPad. Once she was alert and fully mobile, she was allowed to go home. They left the same way they entered the hospital and the HPS let them out of the back door.

The above scenario highlights the need for precise planning and full cooperation with all professionals involved. Had this not been the case the events could have been drastically different. Part of this process includes evaluations and reflection. The mother of this teenage girl said she could not believe how all staff involved worked so well as a team. She had not had any experience of HPSs previously and said she was shocked as she had always thought they simply played with children, which is important, but there is a lot more to the role. She said this experience has completely changed her perspective of the HPS's role. Although developmental, therapeutic and specialised play is a vital part of the HPS role, these are not all of the skills used when working with children and young people with autism. For example:

Preparation and predictability

This teenage girl was able to be prepared via social stories, playing with real medical equipment, and having the school nurse whom she knows well, familiarising her with the blood pressure machine and oximeter. People with autism often appreciate knowing what is going to happen in advance as this reduces anxiety. Individual timetables, social stories, and visual information can help individuals with learning disabilities as well as autism. Pictures, symbols, and Makaton can assist communication and understanding for those who struggle to process verbal communication.

Assisting with sensory needs

"Senses can be processed differently in autistic people. They may find they are over or under sensitive to senses, or both" (Autism Help UK 2021). This is known as hypersensitive and hyposensitive. By gaining this information when carrying out the person-centred assessment and providing reasonable adjustments, the HPS can assist in reducing added stress by reducing noise and touch where possible or familiarising the service user to the feeling (touch) or sound (noise). For example, if a patient requires an ultrasound scan and is sensitive to touch then they are either going to be extremely distressed or very ticklish throughout the procedure. The HPS can desensitise the patient over a period of time prior to the ultrasound, this can be assisted by the family, so that both the HPS and parents are exposing the patient to this type of touch for short periods at a time to the point where they become acceptable to the touch. Once that happens, the patient can then become familiarised to the ultrasound room and the sonographer/doctor who will be preforming the ultrasound scan. When the patient is then comfortable with this process the ultrasound can be performed.

Conclusion

This chapter has provided a snapshot into the HPS's role and given an insight into daily barriers that families and people with autism and/or learning disabilities often face; many of which are related to health and well-being. The importance of teamwork was highlighted as although the HPS in the scenario organised and assisted the patient's admission it would not have gone smoothly without the teamwork and cooperation from all the professionals and family involved. Person-centred care and teamwork should always go hand in hand to provide the best care for our service users.

References

Asperger, H. (1944) Autistic Psychopathy in Childhood (U. Frith translation). In: U. Frith (ed) (1991) *Autism and Asperger Syndrome.* Cambridge: Cambridge University Press

Autism Help UK (2021) What Is the Difference between Hypersensitivity and Hyposensitivity? [Online] Available from: <https://www.autismhelpuk.org.uk/post/what-is-the-difference-between-hypersensitivity-and-hyposensitivity> [Accessed 17 July 2022]

Care Act 2014 (c.23) London: HMSO [Online] Available from: <https://www.legislation. gov.uk/ukpga/2014/23> [Accessed 16 July 2022]

Disability Discrimination Act 1995 (c.50) London: HMSO [Online] Available from: <https://www.legislation.gov.uk/ukpga/1995/50> [Accessed 16 July 2022]

Equality Act 2010 (c.15) London: HMSO [Online] Available from: <https://www.legislation. gov.uk/ukpga/2010/15> [Accessed 16 July 2022]

Health and Care Act 2022 (c.31) London: HMSO [Online] Available from: <https:// www.legislation.gov.uk/ukpga/2022/31 [Accessed 16 July 2022]

Hogg, C. (1990) *Quality Management for Children, Play in Hospital.* London: Play in Hospital Liaison Committee

HPSET (2013) *Code of Professional Conduct for Registered Practitioners and Students.* Healthcare Play Specialist Education Trust and National Association of Health Play Specialists. [Online] Available from: <https://hpset.org.uk/HPSET_copc.pdf> [Accessed 16 July 2022]

HPSET (2019) *Health Play Specialist Standards of Proficiency and Professional Standards.* Healthcare Play Specialist Education Trust and National Association of Health Play Specialists. [Online] Available from: <https://hpset.org.uk/HPSET_ps.pdf> [Accessed 16 July 2022]

Kanner, L. (1943) Autistic disturbances of effective contact. *Nervous Child* Vol. 2, pp. 217–250

Kool, R. & Lawver, T. (2010) Play therapy: Considerations and applications for the Practitioner. *Psychiatry (Edgmont)* Vol. 7 (10), pp. 19–24

Mencap (2022) *The Oliver McGowan Mandatory Training in Learning Disability and Autism Passed into Law.* [Online] Available from: <https://www.mencap.org.uk/press-release/ oliver-mcgowan-mandatory-training-learning-disability-and-autism-passes-law> [Accessed 16 July 2022]

National Autistic Society (2022) *Transforming Lives and Changing Attitudes.* [Online] Available from: <autism.org.uk> [Accessed 15 July 2022]

NINDS (2022) *Autism Spectrum Disorder Fact Sheet. National Institute of Neurological Disorders and Stroke.* [Online] Available from: <ninds.nih.gov/health-information/patient-caregiver-education/fact-sheets/autism-spectrum-disorder-fact-sheet?> [Accessed 15 July 2022]

Pratt, K., Baird, G. & Gringras, P. (2012) Ensuring successful admission to hospital for young people with learning difficulties, autism and challenging behaviour: A continuous quality improvement and change management programme. *Child: Care Health and Development* Vol. 38 (6), pp. 789–797

Walker, J. (2006) *Play for Health: Delivering and Auditing Quality in Hospital Play Services.* London: National Association of Hospital Play Specialists

Wing, L. (1996) *The Autistic Spectrum: A Guide for Parents and Professionals.* London: Constable

Wing, L. & Gould, J. (1979) Severe impairments of social interaction and associated abnormalities in children: Epidemiology and classification. *Journal of Autism and Development Disorders* Vol. 9, pp. 11–29

15

VIRTUAL REALITY

The new distraction therapy?

Tracey Martin – Health Play Specialist

Virtual reality (VR) is the gaming experience that allows the user to be completely immersed in a virtual world whilst they play. So immersed that they are unaware of how funny they actually look as they fight off a Zombie only they can see; funny that is, until they send a favourite vase crashing to the floor! So just how immersive is it? Enough to forget you are having a painful procedure whilst you play? This was one of the questions I was hoping to help answer in the Summer of 2021 when I started a full-time, six-month research study entitled *Virtual Reality Distraction Therapy (VRDT) During Painful Procedures.*

However, this chapter is not about the data and results of our study, but about sharing my experience of using VR headsets with patients aged 8–18 years, so that others might learn from it (Figure 15.1).

Background

At the time of starting our study there had already been a number of small studies conducted on the use of VR, mainly within oncology, dentistry and the treatment of burns. The number of UK-based paediatric studies was limited and with small numbers of participants. Eijlers, R. et al. (2019) carried out a systematic review of existing studies specific to patients aged up to 21 years. They concluded that VR is an effective distraction intervention in reducing pain and anxiety in paediatric patients undergoing a wide variety of medical procedures. This was confirmed by one of the major findings of our study:

> Children and young people predominantly reported feeling more happy, relaxed and confident when using VR, rather than anxious, worried and afraid about treatment.

Gulyurtlu et al. (2022, p. 17)

DOI: 10.4324/9781003255444-19

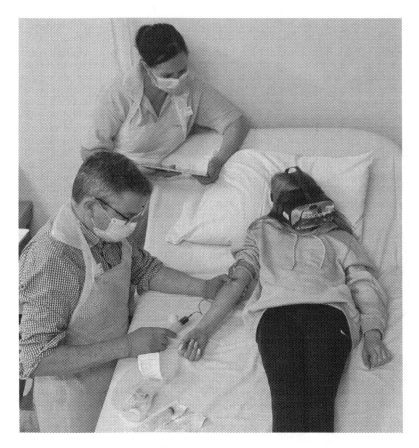

FIGURE 15.1 Virtual reality headset in use during a procedure.

Eijlers, R. et al. (2019) describe VR as being "a fully immersive 3D environment displayed in surround telescopic vision on a head-mounted display" (p. 1344). Full immersion is described as the user feeling as though they are present in the virtual environment. They suggest the use of fully immersive VR is related to pain reduction because the user has less attention available for pain perception.

At the time of writing, my VR experience is predominantly with patients during a painful procedure, but I am also aware of the wider and varied potential for VR use in hospitals. There is scope for developments in many other therapies and condition-specific treatments. For example, encouraging movement necessary for rehabilitation and physiotherapy, using tailor-designed games on the headset, could make sessions more fun and increase cooperation with otherwise tedious and repetitive movements.

Before starting the research post I had used relaxation/mindfulness apps on the VR headset with a young person struggling with anxiety and an eating disorder. She was in hospital for a long period of time and her mental well-being was improved with her ability to transport herself virtually out of the four walls of her hospital cubicle. When she was feeling overwhelmed she would sit at the side of a forest stream or follow some of the mindfulness breathing exercises to relax and calm herself. The immersive and soothing nature of VR could be useful in so many other situations with children and young people (CYP) and may also help as an additional therapy for patients struggling with chronic pain.

Relaxation apps were also used in the study, helping to relax patients before and during the procedure. They were useful as an easy user-friendly option, suitable for patients of all abilities, who wanted to experience VR but for various reasons were unable to operate a game. Although the games were specifically designed to be playable whilst sitting still for a procedure, the use of sedation for procedures such as rheumatology injections generally makes patients too sleepy to operate games. Also, it is apparently very difficult to coordinate inhaling Entonox (gas and air) through a mouthpiece at the same time as trying to dodge missiles and rescue cows from alien abductors!

Advantage or disadvantage?

> One of the main advantages over other methods of distraction therapy is that the child/young person using a VR headset cannot see the procedure.

When using, e.g., a *Where's Wally?* Book, there is always the possibility the patient will catch a sneaky glimpse no matter how well positioned that book is. Whether it is a patient who becomes distressed at the sight of blood/needles, or one who simply prefers to look the other way, the VR headset is the perfect choice as it covers their eyes. I found it particularly useful for dressing changes on injuries the patients would rather not see until it was healed.

> One of the main disadvantages over other methods of distraction therapy is that the child/young person using a VR headset cannot see the procedure.

There are some CYP who just need to look at what is happening to them. Over the years I have witnessed well-intentioned staff positioning the *Where's Wally?* book over a protesting child's arm to block their view of the procedure. The longer the book is held in place the more distressed they become, only calming and cooperating when the book is removed. The same applies to the headset, but instead of a book blocking their view they have something physically covering their eyes. I have met some patients who have decided against using the VR headset based on that need to look at the procedure. Others have tried it after being reassured they can remove the headset at any time.

Reasons for needing to look include:

- Knowing when to expect the pain
- To see if the procedure is going to plan
- To check they aren't being tricked and nothing else is happening
- To know when it's over
- To be involved and have a sense of control of the procedure

The need to look is not exclusive to CYP who are nervous about the procedure. For some, watching is part of their coping strategy and even the most confident patients can become anxious if we try to change that. Patients should therefore be thoroughly prepared, not only for the procedure but also for the VR experience. This will enable them to make an informed choice about whether VR distraction is suitable for them. I understand that a VR training manual for play staff is likely to be available on Starlight's website. It offers tips and advice on preparing CYP and how to assess them for suitability for VR use.

Patient experience

During the study there have been some instances where the use of VR has made a massive difference to patient experience. But one day during the study, I reflected on one uneventful morning and the seemingly insignificant experiences of three patients, all aged 14 years, all using VR during cannulation.

Patient 1: Admitted for the first of many regular IV infusions. She was nervous, requiring topical anaesthetic cream.

Outcome: She had a positive first experience, helping to reduce anxiety for the next visit.

Patient 2: Regular attender, uses cold spray and copes by holding Mum's hand and burying his head in her so as not to see.

Outcome: Coped with the procedure sat upright and without any physical contact from Mum.

Patient 3: Regular attender, copes by watching the needle go in and then looks away. She insisted she had to look so I explained VR was probably not for her but she decided as long as she was told when to expect the needle she wanted to try.

Outcome: Didn't remove the headset to look because she was so distracted by the VR for two attempts.

All three patients used VR for the entire procedure, all were happy, engrossed and having fun. To an observer it would probably have looked like an unnecessary morning in the world of VR. No drama, no tears, all older patients who clearly didn't need any distraction anyway. In fact, despite none of these distractions having an obvious wow factor, each patient positively benefitted from VRDT in a different way. Those benefits may look small and insignificant to us, but for those patients, their personal achievements were huge.

Since recently completing the study, Starlight extended funding for my role, to continue providing VR at Leeds Children's Hospital, whilst testing a different VR kit. Previous study participants were then allowed to use VR again. This opened up a whole new interesting area of the effectiveness of repeat use. Would the novelty of VR fade? Or would continue use build an increase in effectiveness?

At the time of writing I have seen some regular patients three or four times, who were having cannulas sited ready for an IV infusion. There is a group of these patients who are anxious before they come to hospital, wondering if VR will be available that day. They are instantly relieved and reassured, going on to have another positive experience. They tell me of bad experiences when VR wasn't available, of multiple failed attempts which were traumatic and upsetting. Yet I have seen the same patients go on to be oblivious to how many attempts there were whilst they tried to beat the VR game current high score. In fact, the longer the procedure takes, the longer they get to try! I have even had patients say they would have another cannula if they got to play longer! There are also multiple patients, like patient 1 (above), who used VR on their first visit and then returned on their 2nd visit confident because they knew they could cope with the procedure. Patient 2 can now have his cannula without an accompanying parent's support, with or without VR. Another patient now has his cannula without numbing cream after trying with the VR first.

Seeing children walk excitedly to the treatment room for their procedure, with the VR foremost in their mind is fantastic. Even some of the nervous children are more easily treatable with the help of the VR. Reassurance that they are just trying out the VR first, no tricks, allows them the confidence to try a game. Concentrating on a game helps to reduce the usual build-up of anxiety by keeping medical equipment out of sight and out of mind. Once they are happy and playing, being told the procedure is starting often doesn't seem as bad as it did before. Patient delaying tactics, exacerbated by watching are minimised as a result.

Of course, VRDT is not suitable for every individual, procedure or situation. Although there have been some amazing exceptions, most CYP who need to look or who have a severe procedural anxiety are not going to be persuaded to wear a headset and ignore what is really happening if it scares them. Could this be achieved over time by including VR in desensitisation sessions? Can we reduce the need for a general anaesthetic as a last resort by providing a fun new coping strategy? Will using VRDT routinely with children early in their hospital journey, alongside play preparation, help to prevent some of those anxieties from developing in the first place? Why are some children unable to switch their focus from the procedure, whilst other usually anxious patients are totally immersed in another world? VR use in hospitals is still in its infancy so we don't yet have the answers to all these questions. I for one, can't wait to find out!

Acknowledgements

Dr Alexander Paes, Paediatric Respiratory Consultant, Leeds Teaching Hospitals NHS Trust – Chief Investigator

Karl Ward, Lead Nurse for Research and Innovation (Education), Leeds Research and Innovation Academy, Leeds Teaching Hospitals NHS Trust – Chief Investigator

Lisa Beaumont, Therapeutic & Specialised Play Manager, Leeds Teaching Hospitals NHS Trust – Principal Investigator

Starlight Children's Charity – who funded my six-month secondment for this research post

R&I, Leeds Teaching Hospitals NHS Trust

Heather Rostron, Senior Research Nurse, Leeds Teaching Hospitals NHS Trust

Leeds Children's Hospital Research Team

Dubit Limited – for the generous donation of high quality VR headsets used for the research

This research was also funded by the National Institute for Health & Care Research (NIHR) Yorkshire and Humber Patient Safety Translational Research Centre (NIHR Yorkshire and Humber PSTRC). The views expressed in this article are those of the author and not necessarily those of the NIHR or the Department of Health and Social Care.

References

Eijlers, R. et al. (2019) Systematic Review & Meta-Analysis of VR in Pediatrics: Effects on Pain & Anxiety. *Anesthesia & Analgesia*, 129 (S), pp. 1344–1353

Gulyurtlu, S., Martin, T., Paes, A., Beaumont, L. & Robertson, S. (2022) *Virtual Reality Distraction Therapy Report*. London: Starlight Children's Foundation and Leeds Children's Hospital Publication. [Online] Available from: <https://www.starlight.org.uk/wp-content/uploads/2022/06/Starlight_VRDTReport.pdf> [Accessed 22 July 2022]

16

THE ROLE OF THE HEALTH PLAY SPECIALIST IN THE CARE OF CHILDREN AND YOUNG PEOPLE WITH CANCER

Penelope Hart-Spencer – Registered Health Play Specialist

Introduction

The role of a health play specialist working with children and young people with cancer is one that requires skill, compassion, and resilience. It is the most fulfilling and heart-warming, yet sometimes, heart-wrenching role to work within. A diagnosis of cancer is devastating at any age and children, young people, and their families require expert support and holistic care to help them navigate their way through their cancer care journey. Health play specialists working in a cancer care setting need to be multifaceted in their skill base and approach.

As a health professional, it is difficult to comprehend what it must be like for a family when their child is diagnosed with cancer. We understand it will have a tremendous impact on the whole family and will change everything in their lives from the moment their child is diagnosed. We can help them, but we will never know how it feels on a personal level. Each family in our care will have different levels of need and we must be responsive to this. The differences are based on their lived experience, their culture and often informed by their previous health-care experiences. We must consider the cultural needs of our patients and ensure these are addressed sensitively, without assumption or prejudice.

Within our role, we need to be able to work with children and young people within a wide age range (0–18) and understand the families in our care will come from a diverse range of backgrounds and family types. Families with a child with cancer have the difficulty of trying to manage their lives outside of the hospital, with their existing responsibilities. This is particularly difficult if they have children at home as well as a child in hospital. It is our responsibility to ensure we build a good professional rapport with the families in our care, so they feel secure and well supported during a time when they are most vulnerable.

DOI: 10.4324/9781003255444-20

The role of the health play specialist is an integral role within the wider multi-disciplinary team caring for children with cancer. Children who are diagnosed with cancer find themselves in an unusual situation which takes them away from their normal daily routine, often resulting in feelings of unease and worry. These feelings can be alleviated by a skilled health play specialist. Play and recreation must be facilitated as a priority when children are in hospital. We know from experience and research that play is important to children's holistic development and is a universal right under article 31 of the United Nations Convention on the Rights of the Child (Tonkin, 2014). It is essential that children with cancer are given time and space to express themselves playfully and creatively to help them process their experiences, and it is recommended within the NICE guidelines (2021) that children and young people in hospital should be offered sources of support such as a health play specialist.

Incidence of childhood cancer

In the UK, around 1,800 children are diagnosed with cancer each year (Children with Cancer UK, 2022), and the types of cancer that affect children differ from those affecting adults. The most common type of childhood cancer is leukaemia, followed by brain and spinal tumours. These combined make up over 50% of all childhood cancers (Children's Cancer and Leukaemia Group 2022).

Communication

Children with cancer require specialist treatment and care and will be referred to a hospital which has a dedicated oncology ward or unit with consultant paediatric oncologists leading the care. It is a good practice to ask families in our care what is important to them within their healthcare journey. Some wards and day units have 'What Matters to Me' displays, which is an open communication tool to allow children and families to state things of importance and give their opinions about the service. This method of patient engagement is a good way to gain service user feedback, which can be incorporated into the service for patient benefit. Communication is vital and health play specialists can assess and learn about the children in our care and can share important information with the wider team, which will help to streamline their care. This can include information about the child's phobias, preferences during clinical procedures, and any issues that are affecting the child or family. Information should be documented in the patient's hospital record, according to the service policy, so it can be accessed by all health professionals working with the child.

Building trust

Prior to a child being diagnosed with cancer, they will usually have met several health professionals and had lots of investigations prior to being admitted to the oncology ward to start their treatment. Unfortunately, this is often a time of overwhelming stress and strain on families, and barriers in communication and trust issues can build up. There may have been a delay in reaching a diagnosis, and this can prompt feelings of guilt and anger in families. We must remember that families in an oncology setting are often experiencing a wave of different emotions on a daily basis and to alleviate some of this, it is important that children and families learn who they can turn to for support, with the health play specialist often providing lots of emotional and procedural support. It is best practice for the health play specialist to be part of the child's treatment journey from the beginning of their admission and this will help to inform the best approach for the child, which can be shared with the wider team, to promote continuity in care for the child. Research suggests that when children do not have positive experiences of healthcare, it can lead to problems that affect future care, including mistrust in healthcare professionals and increased anxiety about procedures, as cited in NICE guidelines (2021, p. 6). Children who are diagnosed with cancer will be on long-term follow-up for many years and it is important we build their confidence in healthcare from the beginning.

Clinical procedures in cancer care

Cancer care is a very specialist area which involves different investigations, procedures, and treatments. Therefore, it is important that health play specialists working in cancer care learn about the treatment pathways and interventions to plan support which children may require. Cancer care is very complex, and at times, may feel overwhelming. It is important to remember that the role of the health play specialist is not to be clinical or give medical advice to families. We are here to prepare and support children for and during clinical procedures and offer guidance on how best to cope. Some procedures may be painful or difficult for children and their parents or carers may need support during these times too.

When a child is diagnosed with cancer, the types of treatment options may include one or more of the following – chemotherapy, surgery, and radiotherapy. To enable chemotherapy to be given, children are often required to have a central venous catheter (CVC) which can be a Hickman line, PICC line, or Portacath. The CVC is inserted into the child's chest under general anaesthetic to enable access for when the child requires intravenous medications or transfusions. It is important to identify if this is the first time the child has required an anaesthetic. They will need specialised play preparation for going to theatre and an opportunity to explore what they may see, feel, and hear before their anaesthetic. Once a child has a CVC, the need for peripheral cannulation is minimised, which is a positive aspect of the CVC, as many children dislike having needles and cannulas as it is often painful.

A decision will be made by the clinical team as to which device is most appropriate for the child or young person. Where possible, health play specialists should advocate for children and young people to be involved in the decision-making about which device they will have, as it will become part of their identity for the period of time they are on treatment and enables them to feel a sense of autonomy and control. Anecdotally, many young people report a preference of a Portacath as it is placed underneath the skin and not visible. However, Portacaths are not always suitable for children and young people who have needle phobia, as a gripper needle is required to access the Portacath. The pros and cons of each CVC should be discussed to allow them to make an informed decision.

It is essential that children and young people are prepared for any clinical intervention or procedure using therapeutic and specialised play techniques by a trained health play specialist. In practice, preparation for CVC insertion with younger children would include using specialised play equipment including a doll with a Hickman line to allow children to explore the line and see where it may be placed. We use syringes and saline to show children how the lines are used. Familiarisation with real medical equipment helps to desensitise children to the clinical equipment and participating in an experiential learning opportunity, promotes normalisation of the central line for the child.

In some paediatric cancer care settings, children are given their own 'Olly The Brave' teddy which is a lion with a central line and a removable mane. We use this resource when teaching children about central lines and hair loss, which is a side effect of chemotherapy treatment. These are gifted by the charity Molly Ollys Wishes (2020). We also implement the Beads of Courage programme, funded by Children with Cancer UK, which is a bead collection programme and results in a visual representation of the child's cancer journey.

Side effects of treatment

One of the most common side effects of chemotherapy treatment is hair loss. For many children and young people, the prospect of losing their hair is very upsetting and they must be given support to cope with this prior to their hair loss. Some children and young people choose to have a wig, and many are kindly donated by the Little Princess Trust charity. It can help children to cut long hair shorter prior to losing it, and some prefer to remove their hair before it starts to fall out. Directed play can be helpful with younger children to explore feelings connected to hair loss and the use of ribbons, string or dolls with long hair which can be cut or removed is useful in therapeutic play sessions. Age-appropriate literature produced by Children's Cancer and Leukaemia Group (CCLG) surrounding hair loss and other side effects of treatment are available and are a good resource to have.

Children and young people experience lots of changes to their physical appearance during treatment for cancer, which can affect their self-esteem and confidence. Health play specialists can facilitate emotional support to help them cope with these changes and help them to rebuild their confidence as good communication surrounding the thoughts and feelings of the child or young person is essential when exploring their difficulties. Health play specialists may facilitate support for parents, carers, and siblings to help them understand how the child or young person is feeling, and this promotes a very family-centred approach.

Promoting positive experiences

The health play specialist role in cancer care is extremely multifaceted. Each day is different in an oncology setting and you are required to use a range of skills as the role is continually challenging and pushes you to create new ideas for therapeutic and specialised play for patients in your care. It is essential that the remit of the role is conducted in line with the Healthcare Play Specialist Education Trust (HPSET 2019a & 2019b) and National Association of Health Play Specialists (NAHPS 2022) standards and code of professional conduct that our profession adheres to.

The focus of the health play specialist should be to make the experience of being in hospital the best it can possibly be by tailoring play and support to meet the age and stage of development of each child in their care. Their experience in hospital should be playful and include things that children and young people will enjoy and help normalise being in hospital (HPSET 2022). This can include music, games, imaginative, creative, and messy play. Some children with cancer will need play provision on a one-to-one basis if they are in isolation or unable to leave their bed space due to feeling unwell. Chemotherapy can make some children feel very drained and nauseous, so less energetic activities such as story-telling or arts and crafts may be suitable during these times.

When families find themselves in an oncology ward or unit with their child, it is a place they would never wish to be and a treatment journey they never imagined they would be embarking on. No matter what the outcome of the treatment, children and families in hospital should have the opportunity to make memories and always remember their time as a playful and well-supported experience, facilitated by a skilled health play specialist and team of health professionals. It is a privilege to be part of a child's cancer journey, knowing that your skills and care during their time in hospital helped them to understand, feel safe and be themselves, and not just a 'patient'.

References

Children with Cancer UK (2022) *Children with Cancer UK. Helping Children and Young People with Cancer Ring the Bell.* [Online] Available from: <https://www.children-withcancer.org.uk/childhood-cancer-info/coping-with-cancer/beads-of-courage/> (Accessed 20.06.2022)

Children's Cancer and Leukaemia Group (2022) *The Experts in Childhood Cancer.* [Online] Available from: <https://www.cclg.org.uk> (Accessed 02.06.2022)

HPSET (2019a) *Health Play Specialist: Standards of Proficiency and Professional Standards.* [Online] Available from: <https://hpset.org.uk/HPSET_ps.pdf (Accessed 9.12.22)

HPSET (2019b) *Code of Professional Conduct for Practitioners and Students.* [Online] Available from: <https://hpset.org.uk/HPSET_copc.pdf> (Accessed 9.12.22)

HPSET (2022) *What Is a Health Play Specialist (HPS).* [Online] Available from: <https://hpset.org.uk/training-entry/> (Accessed 20.06.2022)

Molly Olly's Wishes (2020) *Supporting Children with Life Threatening Illnesses and Their Families.* [Online] Available from: <https://mollyolly.co.uk/> (Accessed 20.06.2022)

NAHPS (2022) *National Association of Health Play Specialists: Training, Qualifying and Registration.* [Online] Available from: <https://www.nahps.org.uk/hpset-nahps-joint-work/training/> (Accessed 02.07.2022)

National Institute of Clinical Excellence (2021) *Babies, Children and Young People's Experience of Healthcare NICE Guideline.* [Online] Available from: <https://www.nice.org.uk/guidance/ng204> (Accessed 02.05.2022)

Tonkin, A. (2014) *The Provision of Play in Health Service Delivery.* Fulfilling Children's Rights Under Article 31 of the United Nations Convention on the Rights of the Child. [Online] Available from: <https://www.england.nhs.uk/6cs/wp-content/uploads/sites/25/2015/03/nahps-full-report.pdf> (Accessed 18.07.2022)

17

TEENAGERS IN HOSPITAL

Nicky Everett – Youth Support Co-ordinator
Sarah Dransfield – Teenage Cancer Patient

Sarah and I have known each for over 10 years now. I was the Youth Support Coordinator (YSC) on the Teenage Cancer Unit and Sarah was a 16-year-old patient at the time. This chapter is structured around a question-and-answer session between the two of us, we both thought it would be interesting to hear about life in hospital for a young person from the perspective of both sides ... the patient – Sarah and a member of staff – Nicky (Figure 17.1).

Sarah interviewed by Nicky

Q1. What was life like for you as a teenager, prior to your cancer diagnosis?

Prior to my cancer diagnosis I was a 'normal' teenager. Life was what I would describe as 'normal'. I was quite a shy teenager; I did not have lots of confidence in myself, but I had lots of friends and was enjoying going to college. I grew up in a lovely village and spent a lot of time on my grandparent's farm as a child. I had never been poorly in my life, and I used to picture myself living to 100.

Q2. When did you realise something was wrong?

I first realised something was wrong in early January 2012. My family and I had just been away to Thailand for Christmas and as I stepped off the plane, I felt a pain in my knee. I turned to my dad and said that my leg was hurting, and he thought I had just been sat funny. A few weeks went by and the pain in my leg was increasing. By the end of February, I remember being in that much pain, that whilst waiting for the college bus, I had to ask other people to get up so that I could sit down. I was taking painkillers all round the clock and I remember my grandma saying to me, "you should go to the doctors". Whilst at the appointment the doctor told me that he thought I

DOI: 10.4324/9781003255444-21

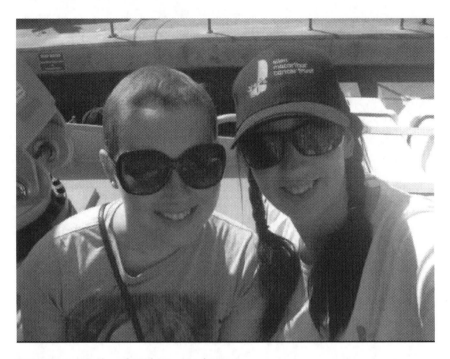

FIGURE 17.1 Sarah and Nicky in sunglasses.

had somehow sprained my knee. He advised me to keep taking the pain-killers and if the pain hadn't reduced in a couple of weeks then come back to see him. That day never came. In the meantime, I went to see a family friend, who was a physio, he knew straight away that something wasn't right. He noticed that my knee had turned inwards. He initially thought that I'd had such a fast growth spurt, that it had caused my bone to move. I started wearing insoles in my trainers, but the pain wasn't reducing and in fact was getting a lot worse. The following week I popped in to see him again and he knew at this point, something was seriously wrong. My knee was now warm and behind my kneecap it felt like gristle and very different to my other leg. I was lucky that he had some great contacts and he booked me in for an MRI scan the next day.

At the MRI scan, I knew something wasn't right, they didn't complete the full scan and gave me the photos to drop off to my physio. The next day the physio rang mum to tell her the awful news that I had got bone cancer. I went for an X-ray that afternoon to confirm what had been seen on the MRI and then went to the doctors. When they told me I burst into tears and asked, "Am I going to die?" Months into my diagnosis, I found out that I had in fact had the cancer growing inside of me for the last six months, so three months before I was even aware of any pain, that was a shock!

Q3. What were you first impressions when you were admitted to hospital?

The first time I had ever stepped foot in a hospital was only a week after I was told about my cancer diagnosis. We had to travel down to Birmingham Royal Orthopaedic to have a biopsy. This was for the doctors to determine which kind of bone cancer I had. At this point I was made aware of the treatment I would be having. Up until then, I had no idea if I was going to even need treatment. After my biopsy and the first ever operation of my life, the doctors sent us back home to wait for the results. I remember the moment we received the phone call to say I had Osteosarcoma. To me at that moment in time it meant nothing. I had never heard of it before. But I was soon to find out the real extent of this disease.

The following day me, my mum and my dad went over to Leeds to discuss my treatment. My first impression of the Outpatients Ward was that I seemed to be the oldest there. We sat in a room with many young and poorly children until we were called in to talk to the doctors. This was where I met my consultant Adam Glazer and my specialist nurse, Sally Burnell. They told me I would be having a very intense chemotherapy regime that would make me very sick, which they would treat with anti-sickness medication; that I would lose my hair; and that it could potentially affect my fertility later in life. They also explained to me that they were going to try and save my leg by replacing the bone with metal, but we would have to see how my tumour reacted to the chemotherapy. To me, what stood out more than anything else was that I was going to lose my hair. Being only 16 my hair meant everything to me. I was devastated. They told me that not one person who had received this treatment in the past had ever managed to keep their hair. This was going to be tough. At that moment in time my fertility wasn't the biggest worry of mine, however, they did give me the option to store some of my eggs for future use but said it would be a much better idea to start chemotherapy in order to save my life. I remember thinking at the time, my eggs would be no use if I wasn't here, so let's just start the chemotherapy.

After this conversation, they took me down to the ward where I would be having my treatment. The first young person that I saw was a young lad in a wheelchair, he had no hair, his face was bright red, but he smiled and said hello. I cried, I thought that was going to be me. I met the nurses and tried to get my head around the fact that this place was going to become my home. I couldn't understand that only a couple of weeks before I was at home living my normal life and suddenly, I was in the middle of a teenage cancer trust unit, about to start fighting for my life. That day I walked onto the ward a healthy girl, I didn't feel like I had cancer, yes, I had a pain in my leg, but the rest of me felt fighting fit. Little did I know, weeks later I would be in a wheelchair struggling to walk, throwing up every 30 minutes, have the energy of a mouse and a year later leaving the ward as an amputee.

Q4. Did you spend any time on either a children's or an adult ward?

The majority of my treatment was on the teenage cancer trust ward for 11 to 16 year olds. With me being 16 and turning 17 midways through my treatment they decided it would be best for me to stay where was familiar to me and not move me to the older teenage ward. However, from time to time I did have to go and spend some time on a children's ward. For example, if they were doing a deep clean of the wards or had run out of beds. I found this very challenging as I had to share a bay with children as young as one year old. They definitely had a different sleeping pattern to me. With being a teenager, I liked to sleep a lot anyway but having my treatment made me extra sleepy, and the little ones used to keep me awake, through no fault of their own. However, it did make me miss the teenage ward. It made me feel extremely thankful to have been given the opportunity to be on a teenage cancer trust ward. Without this, I would have either been on a children's ward or an adult ward; there would have been no in between.

I also spent some time on an adult ward whilst having two separate lung operations. It seemed to me that people were extremely confused as to why I was on a ward with them, as I was so much younger than them. I felt a bit like an alien.

Q5. How did you find treatment, side effects and life in hospital?

I reacted very badly to treatment. The treatment for Osteosarcoma is very harsh and intense due to the nature of the cancer. It was inevitable with the treatment that I was receiving, that I would lose my hair very quickly. This is what scared me the most. I had always loved my long hair, the thought of losing it terrified me. Losing my hair meant I would look poorly and in turn everyone would know that I was poorly. As soon as I started to lose my hair, I had it cut short into a bob to make it more manageable. It was coming out quite fast at this point, so I decided to have it shaved off a week later. I straight away put my wig on so I couldn't see myself bald. That didn't last long though as the treatment made me feel so poorly that my appearance was the last thing on my mind. I was in hospital more often than not and even when I did get to go home I would no doubt be back in the next day for a blood or platelet transfusion. I also got a few infections whilst on treatment which made me extremely poorly. These at times were more dangerous than the actual treatment and would mean I was on antibiotics for days on end. I was very sick, and the nurses told me I was one of the worst sickness cases they had ever seen. They eventually put me on a very strong drug that made me very sleepy and not really aware of what was going on, this was great as I didn't remember much from the treatment and meant I slept through it!

It was decided in about June time that my best chance of survival was to have my right left amputated above the knee. I was devastated. I initially said no "I can't live without my leg" but when I seriously thought about it, I wanted to live so I didn't have much choice.

Q6. Where did you find support to help you through this period of your life?

At first, I didn't take advantage of any support offered to me. I was very unhappy with only recently being diagnosed and I think I was in denial. Cat – the first YSC I met was so lovely and was offering me to join them in the day room, but I never accepted. Somehow, one day I had a change of heart, I thought if I am going to be in here for the long run I should at least try and help myself. So, from then on, I made the effort to go into the day room at least once a day. Some days we had brunch together in the day room, sometimes pizza night and everyday there would be some kind of activity set up to keep us busy. It also meant we were able to mix with other young people in the same position as me; that was so important. With it being a Teenage Cancer Trust ward, there were no set visiting hours, which for me was great, because it gave my friends and family the ability to visit whenever and for as long as possible. On my birthday the day room was decorated, and I had a party with all my family and friends. Yes, I felt poorly and was hooked up to chemotherapy, but these are memories I'll never forget (Figure 17.2).

I met Nicky a few months into my treatment, and she was just as lovely as Cat. They both very quickly became two of my favourite people! When I was coming out the other side of treatment and feeling well enough to do so,

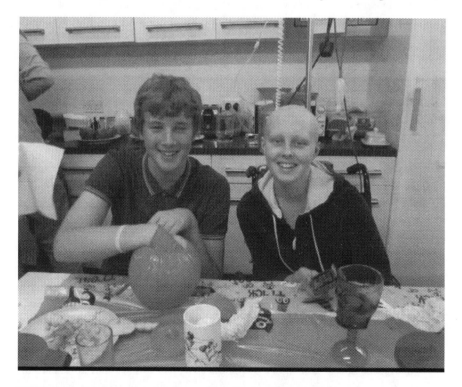

FIGURE 17.2 Sarah and her brother on the ward making pumpkins.

I would join Nicky on trips out with other patients. We went to Flamingo Land, Chester Zoo, Chatsworth House and my favourite of all Find Your Sense of Tumour (FYSOT). This is a conference where once a year, teenagers and young adults with cancer from all over the UK meet up and have the BEST time. We heard talks from a real range of inspirational people, we did activities, we had the chance to talk and open up. Every night we had a party, something a lot of us had missed out on with having cancer in our teens. It was such a confidence boost, but I never wanted to leave.

Q7. How is your life now?
It has taken me a lot of time, but I am now to a point where I am more confident than before cancer or my amputation. It is by no means easy, having to overcome cancer is hard enough without having a new disability to contend with. It took me well over a year to feel confident enough to be able to walk on my prosthetic and even then, I had it covered up to make it look like a real leg. I just wanted to look like a 'normal' 17 year old. My appearance had changed massively, and I didn't feel very happy or like myself for quite a while. A couple of years went by and as I got older, I thought to myself, I should be proud of my leg and what I've been through. So, I booked an appointment with my prosthetist and asked him to remove the foam. I got my metal out for everyone to see and from that day forward it changed my life completely. I am now an ambassador for The Laura Crane Youth Cancer Trust; I have volunteered as a mentor with the Ellen MacArthur Cancer Trust, and I have done many talks in front of professionals about my experiences. I also model for a diverse modelling agency, and I enjoy doing this as I want to normalise disability. I have had many experiences since, that I would never have had the chance to do. I feel richer as a person because I now have a completely different outlook on life that I would never have had before.

Nicky interviewed by Sarah

Q1. If you were to explain your role as a YSC to an alien, how would you do this?How would you explain your role, I never saw you as part of the medical side, you were always the nice part!
The role of the YSC is quite unique. Funded by the Teenage Cancer Trust charity, a YSC looks to support young people during their cancer journey both in hospital and out in the community. There is a focus on two age groups 13–18 years and 18–24 years. The YSC is there to listen, answer any questions that the young people may be struggling to understand or feel unable to talk about in front of their parents/families and sometimes the medical team, all while helping to eliminate isolation during this difficult period.

Cancer doesn't just affect you physically – it can have a huge impact on every other part of your life too. Your Youth Support Coordinator is there to help you deal with that impact and connect with others your age, so you don't feel alone.

Teenage Cancer Trust (2022)

Often it felt like a friendship is built between the young people and the YSC, one of trust and understanding. In my own experience, working as a YSC was one of the most rewarding jobs I've ever had the pleasure of undertaking. I have met and spent time with some incredibly inspiring and brave young people who have battled their journey to the end, one way or another. We are part of the multidisciplinary team (MDT) and we work very closely with the nurses, doctors, physiotherapists, psychologists and other roles within this team. Often if young people had questions or thoughts that they felt unable to share with those around them, we would help them to do this.

Q2. How did you deal with things emotionally?

This is a good question. I think we all have our own ways of dealing with what we see and hear in a hospital setting or out in the community while working within this role. I was lucky in that I had a very supportive team that I could speak to when needed, with the NHS being very stretched and struggling to cope with patient caseloads, there was no input from external teams for supervision and we would often plod along and deal with things ourselves or within our small teams. Taking it home to discuss with our partners/family was not always an option, for one reason – patient confidentiality, but also because family and friends would not understand and should not be expected to.

Our role often involved supporting the families alongside the young person, this was a difficult time for them too and often, like the young people, they would find that friendships became strained due to a lack of understanding and their life now heading in a different direction. Our role can be incredibly varied from one day to the next and some days are much harder than others. For some young people who need end of life support and care, this can be an incredibly difficult time for all those involved The patients are not our family members, but they do become a significant part of your life, and we care about them and the journey they are on.

I remember spending time with a 17-year-old girl who was palliative and being supported at home during this time. Their Macmillan nurse and I had spent a lot of time with the family, and I remember having an afternoon tea in the young girl's bedroom at her home along with her mother, we all sat on her bed enjoying time socially, supporting those final memories, while also helping to distract the young girl from the discomfort she was in. Her mum thanked us for doing this after the young lady had passed away saying it was a lovely memory to cherish from those final days.

Another occasion that I can recall that will always stay with me, was being asked by a family to take hand and footprints from their daughter who had just passed away, as they wanted them for their memory box. I had known this young girl for many years, and I was more than happy to do this for the family, but this was one of the hardest parts of my role. Especially when after doing this and handing these precious prints over to the grieving family, holding back you own tears, I would then go on to introduce myself to a new family coming onto the ward who were looking for reassurance and a friendly face. One day to the next was never the same and it was often an emotional rollercoaster.

Q3. Where did you get your inspiration from, for what to provide for us, for instance, when it was Halloween, you would do Halloween activities, but they would be age appropriate?

This was very patient led and centred. I have worked with children for most of my career prior to working with teens, and providing crafts, messy play and engaging in role play was always an easy go to with these young patients. However, this was very different with young people.

I remember setting up a workshop/project that would run over a number of weeks, where I invited a graphic designer onto the ward to help us individually design some bedding, which would eventually be printed off for the young people to keep. This project started with the young people taking part in a design activity, drawing out ideas for their bedding, this happened by their bedside or in the day room. Then they helped make this come to life on the computer alongside the designer before it was sent off to the printers.

During this project a 16-year-old girl was admitted to the ward, who for the purpose of this we will call Katie. Katie like a lot of young people, came onto the ward looking like a rabbit in headlights and on introducing myself she was very cool towards me and refused to give me any eye contact, that is until I introduced the project I was running. She looked me straight in the eye and said, "bedding … no thank you" in a way where I felt I had just tipped my lunch on her lap!

I spent a number of days and weeks trying to engage with Katie and break down the barriers that she had placed … rather high! I discovered that she quite liked it if I just sat next to her while she was in bed, chatting rubbish. The moment I offered to take her to the dayroom she would shut down. My relationship with Katie became a very close one over the months that she spent in and out of hospital, and me chatting rubbish with her by her bedside became our thing. A good year into her treatment she actually admitted that she wished she had done the bedding activity after all!

Something I did weekly on the ward, which was an activity but probably not seen as one, was a ward breakfast. Every Wednesday I use to do a Tesco shop and buy in some breakfast treats such as croissants, pain au chocolat, fruit, crêpes, fresh juice, etc. All the patients would be told this was happening and more often than not, most of them would get out of bed and come down to the dayroom to have something to eat. They did not need to chat to anyone if they did not want to, but they would listen and feel part of something instead of being cooped up in their room. Often parents would join them too, and it provided a sense of normality again … having breakfast together. For those that normally chose not to be involved in ward activities, this gave me a way in and a time to chat to them and find out a bit more about them and how they were doing, in a very informal way. This would often lead onto me offering them a game of cards like 'Shithead' for example, and this way I managed to get more of a yes out of them than I would just popping my head into their room (Figure 17.3).

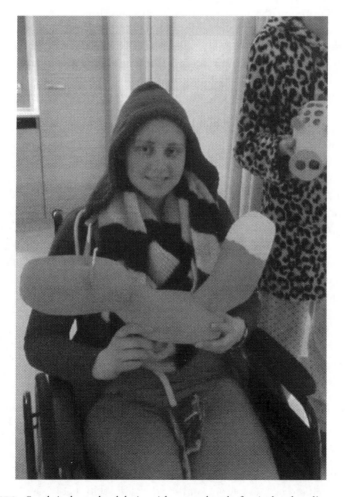

FIGURE 17.3   Sarah in her wheelchair with a wee bottle fox in her hand!

These are just some examples of activities I would provide, the kind of ideas we have for young people and how we engage with them, I would always tailor this to the individual. Sarah, I even remember getting you out of bed while dosed up on ★★★★★ to make 'wee bottle farm animals' out of hospital bed pans and urine bottles, alongside some of the other patients!

Q4. Did you find there was a particular form of distraction/engagement that worked well with teenagers?

Initially with all young people coming onto the ward, there is a period of uncertainty for them and rightly so, they are scared, and suddenly unsure of their future. I have had young people tell me that in those early days of diagnosis everyone approaching them felt like a potential threat. During those early days of induction, for me as a YSC I felt that we needed to be introducing ourselves and spending time with the young people, just as much as the medical team … they needed to know what we could do to help, albeit that help from us was not a cure, but in its own way was part of their treatment and their journey. As I explained with Katie in the last section, the initial meeting and introductions do not always go to plan!

If I am honest, the female patients were more willing to engage with me, whether this was through arts & crafts, puzzles, a chat over a hot chocolate or a bedside catch up. For the boys they often engaged more with me over a game of something like Mario Karts on the XBOX or a board game or my all-time favourite 'Shithead' card game. This was often down to the fact that boys prefer to chat when they are side by side with you, as opposed to sitting face to face.

I remember covering another YSC on the 18- to 24-year-old Oncology Unit, and meeting a young man called Matt who was over 6 ft tall, who mainly came alone to his appointments and actually came across as very confident. However, I quickly learnt that he was scared of small spaces, and he had been told he needed an MRI scan. The only way he would do this was if I would go down to the scan with him, and every now and again hold his hand for reassurance while he was in the machine, he said this helped him cope with being in a small space alone. I did this with him on numerous occasions. It can be the smallest of things needed, but it can make the biggest difference and I think this applies to all age groups.

Q5. Did you have any training to work with teenagers?

This is good question … and no I did not. For some YSC's around the country, they had completed a Youth Work degree, however my background was as a Health Play Specialist (HPS) and I held a degree in Playwork. I started my career working with children from zero through till 18 years. During this time, I found I was drawn to working with the young people and even though this could often be a challenge, for example breaking down barriers, I thrived on this unlike some of the other HPS staff that I knew, who really did not enjoy interacting or working with teens. Personally, I feel you need to have confidence and 'banter' when working with young people especially in this type of setting, as young people want to be treated like young people not children.

With this in mind I did however pick up tips and experience over the years on ways to engage with young people, often these were tried and failed attempts, but it was about not giving up or assuming this meant they were not interested in your support … sometimes young people are just too scared to ask or do not know how.

Reference

Teenage Cancer Trust (2022) *Our Youth Support Coordinators.* [Online] https://www.teenagecancertrust.org/about-us/our-cancer-experts/youth-support-coordinators [Accessed 09.12.22]

18

SHIP-SHAPE AND BRISTOL STANDARD FASHION

The 'Why', the 'What' and the 'How' of implementing the Bristol Standard within the practice of a hospital play team

Julie Fisher – Retired Play Manager and Health Play Specialist

Nicky Bale – Lead Consultant for the Bristol Standard

Jo Caseley – Health Play Specialist

A challenge faced by play teams in the UK is a lack of consistency as to who within NHS Trusts is overseeing the role and the actions of health play teams. Consequently, play teams face having to make it up as they go along, with little or no helpful feedback for their work, good or bad. There is also a likelihood that teams will follow what has always been done rather than feeling supported to make changes to their practice. Team leaders and managers may be restricted by limited budgets – or, in some cases, no budget – for play and a lack of staff. They also face the push-and-pull from higher management, who lack knowledge in the practice of hospital play yet who are the ones to decide if play services in hospital are an essential service they cannot do without, or luxury services they can ill-afford (Webster, 2000; Kennedy, 2010). Broadly speaking, it seems many play teams struggle to find their place within the wider multidisciplinary team (MDT) which is frustrating and can potentially impact staff morale.

Healthcare trusts have found ways to audit and monitor their services, but these are often reliant on both evidence (of which there is very little in the field of healthcare play provision – Tonkin, 2014; Gjaerde et al., 2021) and quantitative figures (they love them!); on everything from patient numbers, admissions and discharges, how long children stay, to what their experience is like when they are here. The value of play in hospital is hard to evidence (Else, 2009) and yet, as Hughes (2001) suggested, play practitioners understand children's play needs in much the same way as a nutritionist understands the nutritional needs of people. Unfortunately for play teams and their managers, play in hospital is

DOI: 10.4324/9781003255444-22

rarely clean, orderly, represented by a nice audit tick box and will not stay sitting quietly on its bed. Structured measurable outcomes within play practices are very hard to find and largely do not exist within today's NHS hospital trusts.

In 2010, Lester and Russell observed:

> The prioritisation of adult agendas in political and economic process can often ride roughshod over children's ability to exercise their right to play, both in everyday life and in extreme circumstances.
>
> *(p. 2)*

In the same way, play teams battle with proving and evidencing the importance of play in hospital even though the work has value and is of great importance to the children, families and to MDT colleagues. One way that play teams can understand themselves better, grow and share the richness of the work, is by learning and developing reflective practice techniques.

The 'Why?'

Julie Fisher, Play Services Manager, Bristol Royal Hospital for Children

The delivery of play in hospital services and the organisation of hospital-based play teams or departments in the UK has no set or agreed format on a national level. This means – in practice – it is difficult for play teams to provide evidence on the impact of their services or evaluate the involvement between play staff and children receiving healthcare. This is an ongoing challenge faced by play service managers.

For hospital play teams, there is no current benchmarking tool to monitor their service provision, no agreed way of documenting their play practice and no widely used method of assessing acuity or patient needs. This differs from other allied health professionals who are members of the MDT, including music therapists, occupational therapists and physiotherapists, even though – like these other professionals – health play specialists (HPS) as individual practitioners are required to undertake a registration process to ensure public and professional accountability.

Both monitoring and improving services is an important part of clinical governance within the NHS. The National Service Framework for Children (NSF) states that evidence-based practice can be "instrumental in achieving high standards of care for children and young people" (Department of Health, 2003, p. 24). However, just as it is very difficult to measure the value of play in many other settings (Else, 2009) it is also very difficult to review, audit and evidence healthcare play services in ways that seem to be more achievable for other areas of healthcare delivery. Once you start trying to show the effects of play in hospital, it is clear that simple – and even, sometimes, complicated – 'tick-box' data collection activities fail to represent the true impact of play staff on children's care.

Having no format to follow for how play teams are organised – or for service delivery and service evaluation – leads to inconsistency within departments and between hospital settings. Without an agreed method, some hospital play teams choose to create their own monitoring or record-keeping systems by which they plan and document play input, hoping it will provide the information required about children receiving play whilst in hospital. These records can be missed by others on the MDT and sometimes, experience suggests, the contribution of play staff may also be overlooked or disregarded by others on the MDT. Both scenarios can impact patient care but can also leave play staff questioning, "What is the point of documenting my work, if other staff groups do not read the notes?" If there was a consistent way for play staff to document their assessments or sessions in patient notes, this would perhaps better represent them to all MDT members involved in the patients' care and provide important information regarding our observations or a plan that has been created to support a child through a procedure.

All this raises the question of how play can have a voice and to make an impact within the administrative systems of the hospital. For play managers and their teams, it can feel as though, fundamentally, play does not fit within hospital structures – even though we also know and believe that play makes a significant difference in how children experience their care and treatment in hospital. The HPS job description calls for the establishment of effective communication with children and families and all members of the MDT and for information to be shared with relevant professionals within the healthcare trust. In practice, however, consistently contributing in these ways and showing the importance and impact of our work can be challenging.

We wanted to be a stronger team, more able to reflect on what we do well and how we can improve. But how could this all be done when play doesn't seem to fit into hospital tick-boxes? As the Play Team Manager at a large city centre children's hospital, I was approached to look at the Bristol Standard as a way to create supporting evidence for our practice and embedding a more reflective team approach.

Looking through the well-organised folder of information, this was clearly what we had been looking for: clear objectives and dimensions which covered the wide range of developmental challenges for children within any environment where they can play and learn.

My initial reaction was "Wow!" – and I did not need to be convinced!

There was a sense of excitement that at last, play in hospital could be delivered and the impact evaluated using this structure. The team could work towards a goal, with opportunities to set objectives and values and space to reflect. Here, there would be accountability for the quality of our work that would be presented to, and scrutinized by, the Bristol Standard validators each year to confirm that the required criteria were being met. Outside of the Healthcare Play Specialist Education Trust (HPSET) registration renewal (required by HPSs as individual practitioners), a structured approach to guide how teams work together to achieve shared goals and objectives did not seem to exist within healthcare.

But would the team agree? Would they accept the challenge, too?

The 'What'?

Nicky Bale, Lead Consultant, The Bristol Standard

The Bristol Standard was originally created in 1996 by a team of multidisciplinary professionals who agreed that they wanted a framework that could be used equally by all Early Years settings in Bristol. It was hoped that the framework would support continuous quality improvement through a dynamic annual cycle of discussion, reflection, self-evaluation and actions. In addition to the Birth to Five framework (for Early Years settings), there is also one for Play Provision and this has been warmly received by the Play sector.

The most effective way to maintain high quality practice and provision is through a cycle of reflecting on what you are currently doing, and identifying what improvements can be made. One of the Quality Improvement Principles, laid out by the National Quality Improvement Network (2013, p. 43) states, "when continuous quality improvement processes are embedded, attitudes of reflection and evaluation underpin ongoing practice development". It is this cycle that is at the heart of the Bristol Standard, a framework that provides childcare, early education and play settings with a tool for self-evaluation and support for continual improvement.

When settings decide to undertake the process for achieving the Bristol Standard, teams are assigned a dedicated mentor who will take them through the process and provide support as required. They also have access to network meetings led by experienced mentors where they can meet other settings on the journey. These are very positive and supportive events where deeply reflective and searching conversations take place. Settings also have access to all the online resources associated with the Bristol Standard such as the 'Outdoor Play and Learning' reflective booklet.

Over the years, the framework has undergone several reviews to keep it up to date with current research and practice. It has stood the test of time and – despite changing Government priorities – has continued to be a mainstay for practitioners. During the global COVID-19 pandemic, practitioners said it was the solidity of the Bristol Standard that kept them grounded in quality and enabled them to maintain strength as a team.

The overarching principles of the Bristol Standard have been mapped to the Quality Improvement Principles (www.bristolearlyyears.org.uk/the-bristol-standard/nqin). These principles are concerned with supporting and facilitating local authorities to enable early years and play settings to improve quality. They were developed by the National Quality Improvement Network of which the Bristol Standard is a member. This group is run by the National Children's Bureau and is a supportive group for strategic quality improvement leaders in local authorities and policymakers. The principles underpin the vision and values of the Bristol Standard framework which consists of ten dimensions of quality that the settings work through over two or three years, depending on which of two pathways they choose to follow (Figure 18.1).

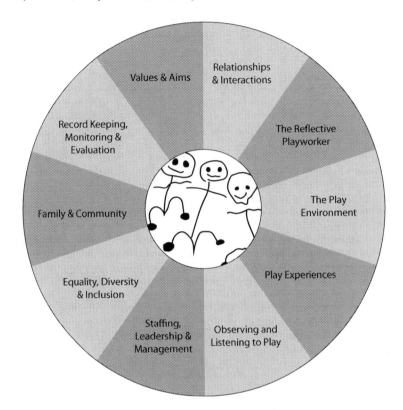

FIGURE 18.1 Bristol Standard for play dimensions wheel.

(From Bristol City Council, 2019, p .3)

The ten dimensions of quality cover every aspect of Early Years and Play:

Encouraging teams to discuss each of these dimensions, identifying what is already being done well and what requires change or improvement is the most effective way to embed the Bristol Standard in development plans and actions for the year. This way it does not present as extra work but rather becomes part of the core work of the setting. Those who use the Bristol Standard to evaluate their setting are passionate about continually developing their knowledge and practice. When teams have completed the process and have had their submission validated, they may display their achievement of the Bristol Standard within their setting, on paperwork and during inspections. Achieving the Bristol Standard has become recognised as an indicator of settings that are committed to consistently improving their practice through self-reflection within Bristol, the surrounding areas and beyond.

A feature of the Bristol Standard is that it is a positive approach, not a deficit model. The process always starts with celebrating what the setting is already doing well – their strengths. This sets teams off on a high as they produce evidence to back up these strengths. As practitioners, we do not always focus on what we do well, and can be quite critical of ourselves, so it is good to have this upbeat focus from the start of the process of change. Settings then identify areas to focus on next which become their targets for the following year. Next comes the important part. Every action must show what the benefits for the children will be. For example, if the target is to make a sensory area in the garden, the team must really think in depth about the impact for the children of what they are planning to develop.

Children are at the heart of the Bristol Standard and by ensuring that settings identify clear benefits for children in their care for each target, it ensures that they keep children at the centre of everything they do. It is encouraging that improvements can be seen easily – sometimes actions are small, and results can be seen straight away, such as labelling all resources to encourage children's independence, while others may be more long term such as a garden development where progress can be seen more gradually.

The strength of the Bristol Standard is that it brings teams together. The reading materials and reflective questions are designed to form the basis of whole team meetings. Everyone within a team is encouraged to have a voice and it is intended to be empowering to all. Young team members who seem too nervous to speak at the beginning of the Bristol Standard journey gain confidence and begin to take on responsibility for actions. The pride in their achievements is evident as their enthusiasm grows.

The Bristol Standard can also provide important supportive spaces for those working alone in their work with young children and families. Childminders have said how by doing the dimensions together in a group they have already talked about the strengths and actions, so in effect have rehearsed any conversations they might need to have with visitors or stakeholders. It gives them a much greater self-confidence and belief in what they do.

The Bristol Standard team is always looking to develop further, supporting teams and developing resources to fit an increasing variety of settings. We are keen to work in collaboration with other professionals. In the most recent editions of the frameworks, we worked with Public Health colleagues to ensure that health matters were woven through the dimensions. We have been particularly excited to work with play teams in hospitals and to give them a framework to help them address the challenges of evaluating and showing what they do. The best aspect of working with a hospital-based play team is that it provides a space for mutual learning between play and early years as well as between education and play staff. Bristol Standard validators have learnt an incredible amount about the very important work play teams undertake with children and their families to make the hospital experience easier. They have felt humbled to read the submissions from Bristol Children's Hospital and to hear the play team talk with such enthusiasm about their work. It has been a very valuable experience for all of us.

And the 'How?'

Jo Caseley, Health Play Specialist, Bristol Royal Hospital for Children

Our team has embraced the reflective practice model that the Bristol Standard has opened up to us, and we are now able to present to the Trust year-on-year what we do, how we do it well and a plan for what we are going to improve on next year and into the future.

The challenge was how to get a diverse team of hospital play professionals on board with adopting the Bristol Standard. Learning how to value and make time for quality reflective practice took some time and inevitably there was some resistance. Initially it was a time-consuming process and the teamwork this required took staff away from the children, young people and families on the wards. However, everything that has the power to improve practice is worth the commitment.

Undertaking the process and completing the annual submission of work needed to achieve the Bristol Standard was a little tricky to appreciate at the start. However, the language and the feel of the work gradually became familiar and now everything we do on the wards and in our team fits somewhere within the ten dimensions of best play practice. In due course, the benefits of regularly reflecting on our collective practice were shared, learned from and put into action. Gaps in the service and challenges were more easily highlighted, targets were set to fix the issues and actions allocated within the team to work on.

The ten-dimension model within the Bristol Standard really helped the team think about the bigger picture of the role of the hospital play team. Whilst working through the dimension about family and community, for example, it highlighted the significant amount of co-working we do with schools, social care teams and local authorities in order to ensure the child's progress through play in hospital can continue after they are discharged.

In practical terms, the play team work on the Bristol Standard in small groups and each group has an equal share of job roles, working hours and banding within the team. This means the groups are able to sustain sharing and achieving workloads and learning from each other. Each year the groups are remixed to ensure all staff benefit from working with different people who have different working practices. This supports more diverse learning and skill sharing.

At the start of the year the whole play team agrees on priority targets and which of the ten dimensions to focus on. The whole team is responsible for supporting these targets. Then, small groups undertake planning for what needs to happen next and share with the whole team on a regular basis to communicate progress, ask for advice and get a collective approach regarding how to move the targets forward. At the end of the year, each group will have completed the reflective writing and supporting evidence to show how the team achieved or made progress with the targets and dimensions.

Evidence is found in all different kinds of formats across the teams' work including Standard Operating Procedures (SOPs) written to reflect the targets met the year before, and photos of new resources or improved play spaces highlighted as being in need of improvement in the previous year. The team have created focused plans for their work with children and young people to improve the play services offered by a self-evaluation process talked about using the different ten dimensions. The beauty of the play standard is that we can only evidence what we have already achieved. Therefore, by improving the service as we work through the play standard each year, we are creating the evidence to show the improvements.

As a group we have achieved some really wonderful whole-team working when setting and achieving the priority targets each year. For example, the dimension covering 'Values and Aims' needed the team to think really hard about who we are as individuals and as a group of professionals, what we do and why. With no clear guidance from the Trust or outside bodies on how to structure our team and deliver our work, this is incredibly hard. The roles within the hospital play team are probably the most varied and misunderstood jobs in the hospital environment. Colleagues see us at work, but there is little to explain or demonstrate our method for working or to account for the 'successes' within our work. A play specialist rarely gets the credit for being the person that so very carefully can convince a seven year old to let a nurse put a tube up their nose and supports them throughout such a distressing procedure. Reflective practice has helped us understand and ground our own practice. This has helped us feel more confident to start explaining our role within the MDT and further afield.

Across the year, through guided group sessions with one small group leading the way, the team created and established our mission statement and agreed some aims for the play service. We now hold our own underlying beliefs about our hospital play team to account as there is a sense of shared ownership over our mission statement and our values. We talked and questioned each other until we were able to agree collectively who we are, what we do and why we do it.

Without the structure of the Bristol Standard process this would have been very difficult and would not have achieved such a clear and positive result. The process has supported the team to become better communicators with each other – listening and reflecting, really talking about issues and showing an ability to consider things from everyone's point of view. The values of the Bristol Standard have encouraged our team to become more time and resource effective by sticking to the planning and aims for our work.

The most important learning done here was the shift in thinking amongst the play team. We now are a team that feel empowered to try things out, challenge how things are done, ask why and why not and seek ways to improve our practice. Our targets range from small things like getting a range of most up to date sensory aids to large long-term work like a complete overhaul of the team's referral procedure. Both are achievable with some action planning and smart thinking; and both are beneficial to children and young people.

Equally when things cannot be changed, if the guidelines, the budget or someone else's way of thinking just cannot be worked around, we can manage this too. The Bristol Standard and our group discussions towards achieving it have helped us to see areas of challenge or weakness within our NHS trust setting that are out of our hands and which we are unable to fix. The value is always in the reflective practice process, the continuous aim to improve what we can, and to identify the numerous ways that together we can achieve those improvements.

Conclusion

The Bristol Standard has clearly had a very positive impact for the Play Team at Bristol Children's Hospital. Ultimately the outcome has been that individual practitioners, and the team as a whole, have found ways to more openly discuss how to improve the play service and outcomes for children and young people. At first introducing and starting the process felt like a huge challenge, even just understanding how to follow the transcript, and then to complete the set dimensions and chosen values within a timescale, was time-consuming and difficult. Some of the team felt overwhelmed and there were times when staff were too busy to meet, contribute or complete documentation. To support this, a meeting plan and work structure was devised that could be flexible. This reassured the team that patients and the play input they needed would always take priority, but that it was still worth taking the risk to take on the Bristol Standard for our hospital play service. With patience, effort and perseverance, a 3rd year of attainment with the Bristol Standard has been achieved.

The team has become more willing to try things and openly question why things happen in play – and within healthcare settings – the way they do. This process has developed times of team reflective practice where individuals feel safe enough to ask questions and are equally very proud to share the good work being done in their frontline encounters with children in hospital. It has been an overwhelming success. Until this point, there was no working method that seemed to be designed for full teams to use together. Annual HPSET re-registration is undertaken by individual HPSs only and there is nothing similar that extends to Play Assistants or other well-qualified, very experienced childcare practitioners within teams. The Bristol Standard brings whole teams together and our growth in so many ways has been the result.

If another hospital play team were to consider undertaking this activity, they would need to start by really reading and understanding what the ten dimensions of play are and to 'see' them in their own setting. Question what each one looks like for your team, and then take time and make a team effort to answer the reflective questions honestly and fully. Consider carefully what is achievable within your team and healthcare trust when setting your targets. Keep expectations realistic – over-estimating what can be done is often when teams start to struggle. The Bristol Standard can be undertaken by any play or childcare setting, but for teams outside the boundaries of Bristol City Council, there is a charge made for the package and the mentoring support that happens alongside the process.

From the point of view of the Bristol Standard validators, it has been an insight for professionals who are largely educationalists to collaborate with a hospital-based play service. It has been enlightening and inspiring and a privilege to work together on the journey to becoming a deeply reflective team. The Bristol Standard has enabled the play team to document their strengths with evidence of all the work they are doing with children and young people. This can now be shared with management teams and outside organisations. The Play Team can now talk knowledgeably about what they do, why they do it and how it is making a difference for children and families. The process has enabled the team to make their work visible and always 'improve on their previous best' – fulfilling the strapline of the Bristol Standard process.

For the future of play, it would be great to see the Bristol Standard being taken up by play teams within hospitals across the UK.

References

Bristol City Council (2019) *The Bristol Standard Quality Improvement Framework for Play Provision*. Bristol: Bristol City Council

Department of Health (2003) *Getting the Right Start: National Service Framework for Children. Standards for Hospital Services*. London: Department of Health.

Else, P. (2009) *The Value of Play*. London: Continuum International Publishing Group

Gjaerde, L., Hybschmann, J., Dybdal, D., Topperzer, M., Schrøder, M., Gibson, J., Ramchandani, P., Ginsberg, E., Ottesen, B., Frandsen, T., and Sørensen, J. (2021) Play Interventions for Paediatric Patients in Hospital: A Scoping Review. *BMJ Open* 11 (7). [Online] Available from: <https://doi.org/10.1136/bmjopen-2021-051957> [Accessed 4 April 2022]

Hughes, B. (2001) *Evolutionary Playwork and Reflective Analytic Practice*. Abingdon: Routledge

Kennedy, I. (2010) *Getting It Right for Children and Young People. Overcoming Cultural Barriers in the NHS so as to Meet Their Needs*. London: Department of Health

Lester, S. and Russell, W. (2010) *Children's Right to Play. An Examination into the Lives of Children Worldwide*. The Hague: Bernard van Leer Foundation. [Online] Available from: <https://www.academia.edu/415484/Lester_S_and_Russell_W_2010_Childrens_right_to_play_An_examination_of_the_importance_of_play_in_the_lives_of_children_world-wide_The_Hague_Bernard_van_Leer_Foundation> [Accessed 26 June 2022]

National Quality Improvement Network (2013) *Quality Improvement Principles, 2nd Edition*. London: National Children's Bureau

Tonkin, A. (2014) *The Provision of Play in Health Service Delivery: Fulfilling Children's Rights under Article 31 of the United Nations Convention on the Rights of the Child. A Literature Review*. London: NHS England. [Online] Available from: <https://www.england.nhs.uk/6cs/wp-content/uploads/sites/25/2015/03/nahps-full-report.pdf> [Accessed 30 June 2022]

Webster, A. (2000) The Facilitating Role of the Play Specialist. *Paediatric Nursing* 12 (7) pp. 24–27

19

MANAGING A PLAY TEAM THROUGH THE COVID CRISIS

Laura Walsh – Head of Play, Starlight Foundation

Resilience is relational and embodied (Braidotti, 2006, 2011) in the staff as well as the children and families; interdependent, rather than something external or independent. So just as the play-orientated interventions of health play specialists (HPS) lift children, young people, and their families, supporting their resilience to the stresses they face, they are more sustainable if those HPS are more resilient themselves. Every time children receive healthcare they must internally transition to, and come to terms with, a new situation (Bridges, 1991); from a familiar way of being to an unfamiliar one. This psychological transition represents a potential threat to their mental health as they strive to cope with the challenge to their sense of a normal and safe world. The impact of COVID-19 pandemic conditions had a significant impact on the elements which support the development of resilience. This piece is written through the lens of direct experience and observations of a children's hospital play team lead during COVID-19; it also draws on available literature for perspective.

Depending on your school of thought, leaders are good if they are strong, unshakable, firm, direct, decisive, etc. During the nascent progress of COVID-19, I was shakable, indeed was shaken. For much of March 2020 (the first month) I had a full-on internal shake, expressing the terror of heightened responsibility for the well-being of a large team, when everything I relied on to be 'normal' was made strange. By April 2020 my eye was twitching for hours at a time, there was no way of predicting what would come next and the illusion of control that we as humans can cling to was gone. I wonder now if I was operating swan-like, seeming calm while paddling furiously under the water or if this was in fact obvious. According to Goleman (2013) leaders direct their focus on their selves (developing self-awareness), focus on others (building relationships through good listening and common ground), and the wider world (perceiving the strategic links and consequences of and connections between things). These modes of giving attention keep

DOI: 10.4324/9781003255444-23

links between the individuals, enhance the team in their practice, and encourage the wider organization to be lively, responsive, and relevant.

Resilience is an important aspect of good mental health. Key elements of resilience, according to Lester and Russell (2008), are the ability to regulate emotions, strong attachment friendships, enjoyment, general positive and optimistic feelings, and being able to cope with stress. It is suggested that play makes a fundamental contribution to all these elements (Lester and Russell, 2008). Play is creation, it warms and softens, opening beyond what is physically there. In play we can manifest other realities, reorder our positions in the world, create new worlds, and play out possibilities. Through playing we try out versions of ourselves, become unstuck, un-isolated, we are connected and infinite, bigger and more powerful, we are creators. The sensory elements of messy play have been connected to the ability to make sense of difficult feelings and safely express anger, providing a release.

Timeline

- 10 March – story in news about a staff member having corona virus
- 15 March – intake of first few patients that are outside of the normal range of conditions from other paediatric settings
- 16 March – change in guidance and press briefings in which the Prime Minister outlines an extensive change in guidance including around coming to work

There was a moment early in the beginning of the pandemic when staff were gathering in our communal office space. News on the beginnings of a serious illness spreading fast across the world and already having an effect in our country, was across all communications platforms. The most recent update was that all 'non-essential' staff should plan to go home and work from there, if possible. There was an unusually substantial number of people from the play team together at once in the room and expressions were nervous, belying the feelings underneath the cavalier laughter, teasing, and banter. I perceived they were here looking for reassurance. The main question being, 'are we essential staff?' To this I was able to answer an unequivocal, yes. It felt good to be able to reassure the team that they were indeed essential and vital staff and a palpable sigh rose from the room. Play teams who were redeployed to other areas of work may have suffered from a loss of purpose which acts as a protective factor, contributing to resilience. An increasing compensatory offer was available for us in the form of donated gifts (hand cream, snacks, meal kits, chocolate, etc.). The message received was that the world wanted to support us and our industrious National Health Service (NHS) bellies and hands.

Timeline

- 18 March – Pret a Manger discounts all items 50% for NHS staff and gives all hot drinks free
- 19 March – London prepares for a lockdown

- 20 March – Dominoes give free pizzas to NHS staff
- 20 March – schools close

In a large team there will naturally be a percentage of the team who have greater vulnerabilities either because of their own conditions or the conditions of those who they live with and care for. For many people, their disabilities are hidden, no one would necessarily be aware as there are no visible features. This inadvertently enables them to 'pass' as those without conditions; this can be both an obstacle and an important aspect of resilience. On 23 March I had finished compiling a list of staff within the team who had specific vulnerabilities, in preparation for redeployment if the situation worsens. To protect those within the team with chronic conditions and therefore extreme vulnerabilities those staff were instructed to leave the site. What then began to unfold was a strategy to keep those staff contributing to the collective purpose of the team as well as supporting them despite their being off site. The main elements are given below.

Careful use of language

The ability of words to shape reality was felt strongly, for example the staff members working at home were referred to in discussions as working from home rather than not in work.

Staying together through communication opportunities

Team WhatsApp chat groups were created, one for the home working group, one for the on-site group, one for the leadership team, groups for small working teams. It gave the team the ability to connect with each other when physically togetherness was not possible.

Connectivity

With the churn and change of location and circumstance it was important to me to be assured that everyone had access to some 1-1 support, someone to check-in with. Throughout the period there were regular Zoom meetings, staff were encouraged to praise each other and praise from other colleagues or families was always shared in the meetings and following notes when it was sent.

Celebrating the positive or funny

This was important to encourage the peak moments that play provides.

Physical activity

Joe Wicks PE was encouraged, as well as walks around the block.

Emotional vents

Sharing feelings, checking in with each other, normalising not being okay, and random acts of kindness were all encouraged.

Timeline

- 2 April – clapping for carers on a Thursday – I wanted to cry, hide, laugh. It brought me a sense of un-realness.
- 3 April – begins the constant placing of flowers around my house, in every room – small arrangements
- 14 April – sowing seeds at home; the team are sharing their creations

Throughout this time the team at home are making and creating art and craft pieces which we shared on social media, as a device to encourage play at home. These activities communicated the power and potential of play for all, but specifically as children were not able to access school. This had the effect of keeping the fire of shared purpose, inspiring creativity, and contributing as much as possible. Remote play sessions were devised using the skilled playworkers at home, to be delivered over Zoom.

Play over the medium of remote video call was a concept I felt the urge to dismiss immediately as impossible. It seemed a priori that if play is connectivity and the way of supporting it utilises subtle cues and tacit knowledge, then play at a distance was not something that could work. When faced with staff, prevented from coming into the clinical environment, and children and young people (CYP) for whom play is more a priority than ever, as the option of visits from family, volunteers, charity partner entertainers all disappeared, all you can do is adapt. The challenges of Wi-Fi, the need for tablets, safeguarding procedures to protect children and staff were tackled and resolved. Play staff devised techniques with sensitivity and openness to the children's play cues that was amazing to observe. The rules of space ad time were bent using matching material and the power of imagination. I once watched a game of hide and seek take place over Zoom in which the child hid in their room for the playworker at home to find. I'm still amazed by that one.

Timeline

- 19 April – my first shoots come up – nasturtiums.
- 28 April – the play team complete and release 'We're All in This Together' a Makaton song in which staff mime and sign along to the song.
- 1 May – self-care strategies appear in the crafts at home: worry tree, worry jar, coping strategies.
- 20 May – delivering remote play sessions continues.

This was at a time when there was no sense of what the worst might look like, no map for where it would go or where it would end. We had no idea of what we could cope with and no idea what we would be asked to carry. A sense of endlessness was most difficult. As play specialists we appreciate the importance of being able to manage uncertainty. However, the size of the uncertainty was oppressive. The lack of things to look forward to began to take its toll; no holidays, evenings out, meeting friends or family, simple pleasures, and moments of connection that we casually took for granted, were sorely missed.

Due to the risk of some staff getting ill and taking large sections of the team with them I took the decision to split the team into two groups and co-locate them. This should have reduced the chance of too many people getting ill at any one time. With different bases the opportunities for incidental interactions severely diminished. The effect of that was damaging, causing a sense of separation and paranoia that was not easily resolved. The noticeable effect of less exposure to others in the team was to increase the stress or rather reduce the protective factors offered by connections. The question of what resilience supporting elements teams can draw on to help them remain bouncy was thought about in detail.

Timeline

- 2 June – 'Stop, reflect, check in, check out' boards are up at the exits, a reminder that these are stressful times and stress can be managed better if it is acknowledged.
- Volunteer peer mentors from within the staff team, were trained by the psychology team to support colleagues.
- Well-being webinars begin – the Play Team host a session to highlight and share their strategies and practices.

My conviction is stronger than ever that to build a formidable team which can survive adversity you need opportunities: to share experiences, play together in some way, feel you are seen and heard, and keep learning and questioning. The deep belly of the pandemic was a crucible that forced me to examine my values, question my assumptions, and hone my judgment. The experience changed me, and it changed the team in fundamental ways.

Much is written about toxic stress, the kind of stress which the body cannot cope with. I am a fan of Brené Brown and in a podcast with the Nagoski twins (Brown 2020) on toxic stress the point was raised that the physical response to stress lasts longer than the stressor. I look back now at the Spring of 2020 onwards and there are blanks, some things I know I could not focus on at the time. I was fuelled by adrenalin; I could not drink coffee much as I was already naturally caffeinated in a way by my body chemistry. I had the kind of mental energy which will help you navigate a disaster; you need to think quickly, not read the small print. The recommendation for completing the stress cycle is: physical activity, breathing, positive social interaction, laughter, affection, a big old cry, and creative expression.

References

Braidotti, R. (2006) 'Posthuman, All Too Human: Towards a New Process Ontology'. *Theory Culture and Society*, 23 (7–8) pp. 197–208

Braidotti, R. (2011) *Nomadic Subjects: Embodiment and Sexual Difference in Contemporary Feminist Theory*, 2nd Edition. New York: Columbia University Press

Bridges, W. (1991) *Managing Transitions: Making the Most of Change*. Reading: Addison-Wesley

Brown, B. (2020) *Burnout and How to Complete the Stress Cycle*. [Podcast] 14 October. Available from: <https://brenebrown.com/podcast/brene-with-emily-and-amelia-na-goski-on-burnout-and-how-to-complete-the-stress-cycle/> [Accessed 29 June 2022]

Goleman, D. (2013) The Focused Leader. *Harvard Business Review*. [Online] Available from: <https://hbr.org/2013/12/the-focused-leader> [Accessed 17 June 2022]

Lester, S. & Russell, W. (2008) *Play for a Change*. London: National Children's Bureau.

Nagoski, E. & Nagoski, A. (2020) *Burnout: Solve Your Stress Cycle*. London: Vermilion

PART IV

Reflections from around the world

20

OH! THE PLACES YOU'LL GO!

A play specialist's journey

Ana Smith – Senior Play Specialist

It's in the middle of my work day.

I receive a phone call from the Intensive Care Unit (ICU) asking for help. Basic details are given over the phone: a woman is currently on life support but she is brain dead and a possible candidate for organ donation.

Her family is with her including her eight- and ten-year-old children.

Can I come and help explain what's happening to her children?

I have often received calls like this. I am a play specialist based in a busy children's emergency department (ED) in South Auckland, New Zealand (NZ). Every time, it is an opportunity to use my skills to reduce emotional trauma in children. While each of these scenarios is unique, the common thread is that they are immeasurably sad and raw with human emotion as a beloved person is nearing the end of their life. This is my professional life, 25 years after my initial formal training.

This chapter gives an insight into my professional journey and the diverse opportunities that have arisen during it. Within the chapter I share stories about some of the remarkable children and young people with whom I've been privileged to work and who have shaped who I am today.

Janine was the child who inspired me to pursue a play specialist career. She had suffered a head injury after a hit and run accident while walking to school. I initially met her whilst volunteering in a hospital play programme and later as a teacher aid as she commenced high school upon discharge. She was truly inspirational and taught me so much about patience, perseverance and determination. Working alongside her cemented my desire to begin a career in the play specialist field and I readied myself for the first step in this journey.

DOI: 10.4324/9781003255444-25

A year later, I arrived in Boston, USA ready to start a post-graduate course in Child Life at Wheelock College. It was a big move for a small-town farm girl from NZ and I started graduate school as a very reserved and naïve young woman. I was living in a city 14,000 kilometres from home with limited funds and no contacts. One of the first classes I attended was centred on play and it was at that point that I realised, my play experiences as a child were very different from my American classmates. My childhood experiences revolved around living and working on a farm – making huts in hay barns, trying to catch eels in streams, spending hours making camps in the bush and helping out with chores on the farm. How was I ever going to translate these experiences into playing with American children in a healthcare environment?

During my studies at Wheelock College, I participated in a 6-week internship programme in London. Having been in the United States for the past 15 months, I was now faced with another change in culture but fortunately it felt much closer to home as the terminology was more familiar to me. The most memorable aspects of this internship were the professional connections I made. I was incredibly lucky to have Dr Richard Thompson coordinating our group and appreciated his generosity in sharing his expertise and wisdom in such a down to earth manner. Another stroke of luck was to be completing an internship at a hospital play programme being led by Judy Walker. Working with Judy taught me how valuable it is to have strong role models and mentors who can guide you down the professional path, through hurdles and opportunities. She continues to inspire and nurture me to this day.

After graduating, I found employment at the University of Chicago Children's Hospital which was to be my work 'home' for the next four and a half years. The south side of Chicago is an ethnically and socio-economically diverse neighbourhood with high levels of crime and deprivation. However, despite being located in a severely deprived area, the hospital was well resourced and respected. My time in Chicago exposed me to scenarios, families, illnesses and conditions that were unique to living in the USA at that time.

Initially, I was responsible for the infant/toddler programme. It was 'baptism by fire' as my experience with this age group, up until this point, had been somewhat limited. I was the lead in coordinating care for patients in this age group spanning the medical wards, ICU and the Burns Unit. The programme was supported by an amazing volunteer group including foster grandparents who would comfort and engage with our youngest patients.

I then moved on to the school-age group which felt a lot more within my comfort zone. Again, we had wonderful volunteers to support the service we provided at bedside and in the playroom. We were fortunate to have unlimited toys, activities and supplies to give away and use with families. Only when I moved back home to NZ, did I appreciate just how fortunate we were financially with the amount of funding for play resources. The playroom was a child's dream with every toy under the sun available as well as an outdoor courtyard area. Occasionally, children would enter the playroom and be so overwhelmed that they were unable to engage in 'play'. In discussions with families, we sometimes discovered that these children's play experiences at home were limited entirely to technology. As some of these parents had limited play experiences themselves, they were unable to role model for their children. However, with a lot of encouragement and support, the children and parents learned how to play.

My final role in Chicago was to establish a new post in the ED which involved some challenging moments. I learned to gently question and change the practice of very experienced nurses who called the shots in the department. I learned the importance of memory-making with families when patients died, made the environment more child friendly and dealt with the use of papoose boards (used to completely immobilise children for procedures for IV lines and bloods). I thrived in amongst the chaos, the unpredictability and the raw human emotion and realised that ED was my 'happy place'.

Rachel was a patient who made a lasting impression while working in Chicago. She had been a normally-developing three-year-old girl who had stopped eating, speaking, walking and breathing on her own. She spent six months in Intensive Care, had a tracheostomy and was eventually diagnosed with Fazio-Londe disease – a rare, progressive neurological disorder that causes paralysis and respiratory failure. During that time, I worked with her and her family to normalise her life in this least child-friendly of environments. With very supportive nursing and medical staff, we achieved small snapshots of normal life that brought joy to her and her family. Initially, she was so weak that I had to 'play' for her at the bedside being guided by her limited facial expressions. As she improved, we set up a play space on the floor beside her cot, planning play activities which were achievable. She gradually became stronger and could start to vocalise her interests and preferences. We set up a 'bath' using a large plastic storage box complete with bubbles and water toys and it was delightful to see the joy on her face when she sat in this for the first time. We introduced a mirror to her bath routine so she could view the changes to her body in a playful, safe way. In winter, we brought a bucket of snow in to her room so she could play with it. As the benefits of her play sessions became more obvious to the multidisciplinary team, they became more flexible in what Rachel was allowed to do. Despite the amount of monitoring and emergency equipment required, there were visits to the main playroom and Rachel was able to participate in the playroom events including trick or treating for Halloween.

In 2001 I returned to NZ and started working at Kidz First Children's Hospital in South Auckland. South Auckland is a melting pot of diversity – socially, ethnically and economically, with the families and staff a reflection of this. I began working in ED and immediately noticed a lack of hierarchy within the staff that had been inherent in the American system. It felt a more level playing field with every person valued for their contribution.

Additionally, I started working as part of the Burns Team and learned one of my most important lessons – the utilisation of the multidisciplinary model. I got to know my nursing colleagues and their practice so well during very long dressing changes that I could predict their next step and use this to prepare the child and parent/caregiver as it was happening. I became very good at 'narrating' procedures – talking through the process out loud, enabling patients and parents to know what was happening and giving the nurses hints if the child/parent was starting to lose coping skills. My role was crucial in keeping a child or young person and their parent calm and engaged so that procedures did not become any more difficult for them. While pain medications play a significant role in helping children deal with these tough situations, the use of coping strategies and alternative focus is also vital.

My play specialist skills and knowledge have been put to use in non-traditional settings as a result of the working relationships developed with my nursing and medical colleagues. I was involved in drug trial studies of the Meningococcal B vaccine. This involved children between 16 and 24 months who all needed three blood tests, approximately 6 weeks apart. My role was essential in supporting the children through each blood test but more importantly, keeping the parents calm and reassured enough that they would return for the follow-up blood test. I found that quite simple interventions made the difference. We used a comfort position for every blood test, focused on keeping the parent calm and used a pop-up toy and bubbles as the only distraction toys because we knew they worked so well.

Another ED contact led me to become involved in a small team that travelled to Sri Lanka after the Indian Ocean earthquake and tsunami in 2004. The team comprised an ED doctor, nurse, midwife and me, and we were prepared, from media reports, for a high number of orphaned children due to the disaster. While our time there was suddenly cut short due to the increasing political violence, I remember interacting with children revolved around the use of bubbles – endless amounts of bubbles streaming in all directions resulting in squeals of delight as they ran, chased and laughed.

A different experience was participating in a ten-day Operation Smile mission to Dujiangyan in China supporting underprivileged children and families while they were waiting for life-changing cleft palate operations. My role involved establishing a play area and preparing children for their surgery which was challenging due to a significant cultural and language barrier. Luckily I was assigned two enthusiastic translators each day that helped construct a simple preparation book for families. We were based in a Chinese hospital and took all our supplies and resources with us including toys, activities, bubbles, books, colouring supplies and a polaroid camera to take 'before' and 'after' surgery photos. Once again, bubbles were a hit with everyone – the universal toy that transcends all ages and cultural boundaries.

I have now been working in the Kidz First ED for nearly 20 years and while the physical environment has remained mostly the same, there have been many changes due to staff turnover. Patient numbers have increased, processes have changed and yet chronic underfunding and staff shortages continue to be issues. My play specialist role has transformed into a job that continues to challenge and stimulate me every day. My ED role goes far beyond just providing play opportunities and utilises my skills and knowledge to help settle, prepare and support patients and their families through their healthcare visit. My typical day might involve talking with a young person who has overdosed on medication, listening to a mother sob about the difficulties in caring for her baby with no support, debriefing with a nursing colleague after a traumatic resuscitation resulting in death, or coordinating a plan to minimise the stress for an autistic child needing to have bloods done.

Since 2020, COVID-19 has played a significant part in changing the ED environment and experience. Infection control has dictated that our play resources are very restricted. Gone are the bubbles – the mainstay of any play specialist – for distracting distressed children particularly when they first arrive at the hospital. It has been challenging to replicate the spontaneity of pure joy and wonder that bubbles often bring. We now have giveaway packs and instead of toys to distract kids during procedures, we are reliant on laminated 'Where's Wally?' sheets, YouTube and a parent's phone. More importantly we are using our voices, words and body language to convey a calming presence despite wearing gowns, masks and goggles. Less of my role is spent providing play opportunities with much more of my time focused on relationship building, not only with the patients and their families but also with the people whom I work with every day. Supporting my colleagues, who have worked tirelessly for the past couple of years and face varying degrees of stressors in their own personal lives, has brought a new focus to my role.

Upon reflection, I feel an immense sense of privilege regarding the work I do. Despite ongoing challenges in the provision of healthcare services for children and young people, there will always be ways in which our skills and knowledge as play specialists can make a significant difference to how children and families cope with healthcare experiences – wherever they live in the world. I can wholeheartedly say I love my job and all the challenging, joyous and unexpected moments it brings each day, and I look forward to whatever the journey brings next.

21

PLAY IN TWO DIFFERENT WAYS

A reflection on play practice in the United Arab Emirates

Gemma Hookins – Play Therapist

Humara Bushra Ashraf – Health Play Specialist

Sara Costa – Certified Therapeutic Recreational Specialist

Introduction

This chapter highlights the successful implementation of different play practices in a children's speciality hospital within the United Arab Emirates (UAE). This new tertiary care facility was opened in 2016, to all nationalities including the local Emirati population. The hospital included a Child Life Centre, which was under the child and adolescent mental health centre of excellence, where Bushra Ashraf, a play specialist, Gemma Hookins, a play therapist, and Sara Costa, a recreational therapist, were designated to provide therapeutic play services to the inpatient and outpatient departments.

We were commissioned to establish the Child Life Centre with our special-ised practices to train and educate staff on how well these practices complement each service provision, providing play opportunities, using therapeutic play to distract and normalise the situation, as well as being the service provider of non-directive play therapy and non-directive and directive recreational ther-apy. This unique service was designed to provide a holistic approach tailored to each patient's needs, as well as for the patients and their families. This also included group and sibling sessions. Our service focused on the multidiscipli-nary approach where the same patient could benefit from each of our specialised practices to aid their healing both within the hospital and in further follow-up sessions in the outpatient clinic.

In this chapter, we describe in the form of a case study the unique roles a health play specialist, play therapist and recreational therapist have when working with our patients. We explore our experiences of how the healthcare practition-ers and patients' families perceived our specialised roles. We explore the difficul-ties we had to overcome, reflect on the many challenges we faced implementing a new service in the United Arab Emirates, and how we took into consideration the cultural differences that impacted our work. Finally, we reflect on how we

DOI: 10.4324/9781003255444-26

managed to overcome these difficulties and educate staff and families on our unique practices.

Setting up

When setting up the Child Life Centre, being such a new service in the UAE, the team found a huge task ahead; however, we overcame this with teamwork and the inner drive to help our patients and provide the best quality service. Most doctors and clinicians in the hospital come from different backgrounds, practices and nationalities, the majority being from Asia. In the beginning, it was evident that the UK and US/Canadian trained healthcare providers were somewhat familiar with health play specialists, but were not aware of play therapy and recreational therapy and how the practices differ. The majority were either not aware and didn't know how or when to implement our service or did not think it was relevant or necessary. It was clear from feedback from some healthcare professionals, such as doctors and nurses, that they felt providing play activities for patients was their role and believed that we were there only to entertain the patients as opposed to providing therapeutic interventions.

The hospital setting is a very intimidating and unfamiliar place for children; therefore, some children will feel anxious and fearful, away from their families, while enduring painful procedures. Coyne (2006) examined children's experience of hospitals and found research exploring how patients can feel scared and anxious. Play is very important for children, Else (2012, p. 81) suggests, "The elements of play are varied: it is something that is often fun, driven by intrinsic motivation, undertaken for its own sake". Play is something that children engage in, which can help relieve boredom, provide a distraction as well as some familiarity. Furthermore, it releases energy and pent up stresses. Therefore, anxiety can be reduced in those children receiving unstructured play activities during their hospitalisation (Yateem et al., 2016).

It was our role to change these attitudes. Therefore, the team developed an action plan, starting by educating the staff. We set up a Child Life Centre awareness campaign, where we worked with our marketing team to produce literature, in-house visuals, such as information displayed on the hospital communication television screens, posters, and social media posts. We were creative in using our playroom set-ups, where we organised events for the patients and daily playtime in the hospital's main play area for patients and their siblings, providing a normalised environment.

Our Child Life Team further developed short videos and child-friendly posters around the hospital to explain our service and the benefits of play. In addition, we provided many presentations and interactive workshops for the healthcare professionals from around all departments within the hospital, to showcase our unique service and how our team could help the patients effectively. Setting up this project was a great success, we started to receive referrals for the correct specialist/ therapist and were also asked to present for other centres of excellence and for external healthcare professionals, which then meant we were able to disseminate information to a wider audience on the benefits of play in hospital, play therapy, play specialists' work and recreational therapist.

Play and its specialities

As the professions of health play specialist, play therapist and recreational therapist are very new concepts in the United Arab Emirates, and the concept of 'play' is not taken seriously. There were a few challenges. It came as a surprise just how challenging it would be and, taking the cultural aspects into consideration, how it would affect the way we worked. There have been a few encounters where caregivers, for example, did not want to engage their child with our service or allow their children to take part, feeling reluctant because this was something new to them.

Inpatients

Within the inpatient setting the parents preferred to stay near their children, so that they were able to observe the interaction. They would ask many questions and often answer for their child, and they believed we were there to teach or entertain, as parents have high expectations for learning, study, and homework. However, as we were establishing a new service, we used this opportunity to educate each family about our approach. It was challenging having only one speciality of health play specialist (HPS), play therapist and recreational therapist covering the inpatient and outpatient departments. Therefore, to meet our patients' needs and facilitate workflow, our colleague Sara Costa, the recreational therapist, created a referral pathway and preliminary assessments with inclusion and exclusion criteria. Our time was spent between in-house interactive training workshops (where we provided hands on sessions for the staff for better understanding of each role), education for parents, distraction and teaching, and therapeutic sessions for the patients. This was well received by all staff and parents, and we followed up each educational session with a set of questions to consolidate what was taught. Feedback from the sessions was positive which helped us to evaluate the effectiveness of the workshops.

Outpatients

For the outpatient clinic, at first, there were many assumptions about our roles, Each practitioner had different colour scrubs with the child life teddy bear logo. However, most of the families would refer to us as 'doctor', which was due to cultural aspects, with most local families referring to all hospital clinicians as doctor. Therefore, time was spent educating parents and professionals alike on our unique roles. Furthermore, as time passed and our service became known, the benefits of our roles within the hospital did not go unnoticed. Healthcare professionals, and families alike, would request our service and always appreciated the intervention. This was acknowledged verbally and from our feedback parent questionnaires. For example, feedback from the family of patient 'A': "the play therapy sessions have helped 'A' to attend the hospital and articulate his feelings about his hospital treatment to the doctors and nurses".

It was noted by the parents and healthcare professionals that when the patients were involved in our activities, they seemed less focused on the procedure as they were engaged in play. Providing what Hubbuck (2009) calls 'normalisation' for the patient benefitted them and further aided normality in a potentially scary environment. For example, a recent study has shown that colouring activities can reduce anxiety in children in a hospital setting (Prasetya, 2021), as the children are distracted and doing something they love.

Play therapy

Play therapy complements the troubled child, as they are using familiar tools that they understand. "Play is a voluntary, intrinsically motivated, child-directed activity involving flexibility of choice in determining how an item is used" (Landreth, 2012, p. 11). It helps them overcome internalised issues within a safe trusting therapeutic environment – for example, helping an anxious child in an unfamiliar environment to regulate their emotions and feel comfortable using play. This is facilitated by a trained therapist who validates and accepts the child as they are, giving them the freedom to lead their play. The therapist does not hurry the therapeutic process; their presence is intended to support and facilitate the session at the child's own pace. As Landreth (2012) mentioned, the success or failure of the therapy rests on the therapeutic relationship. The therapist is non-judgemental and non-interpretive, only setting boundaries to protect the child and the therapist. Play therapy provides the opportunity to solve internalised conflicts and improve self-regulation. Axline (1974) explained that since play is his natural medium for self-expression, the child is given the opportunity to play out his accumulated feelings of tension, frustration, insecurity, aggression, fear, bewilderment, and confusion.

Carl Rogers (1942) developed the client-centred approach to therapy – later in 1951, called the person-centred approach. When applied to play therapy, this approach relies on building a trusting therapeutic relationship with the therapist, and letting the child lead the play. The play therapist's role is as important as the play therapy itself. "The presence of an accepting understanding, friendly therapist in the play-room gives him a sense of security" (Axline, 1974, p. 17). Non-directive play therapy was developed by Virginia Axline, utilising the theoretical foundations of Rogers' (1951) person-centred approach, giving the child the opportunity to lead the session, and relies on the child to heal themselves (Figure 21.1).

Furthermore, the non-directive method gives the individual the opportunity to self-heal, by using toys to communicate a problem, and work through it in a

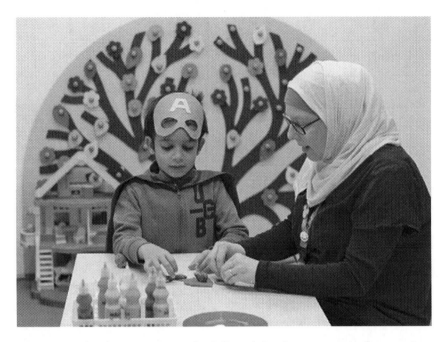

FIGURE 21.1   Play therapy session in the dedicated play therapy room in the outpatients clinic. (Picture taken by our marketing team with a child actor at Al Jalila Children Hospital)

safe setting. Axline herself brought attention to the potential of play therapy with her book *Dibs in Search of Self* (1966), which offers an introduction to the use of non-directive play therapy to solve internalised psychological issues. Play therapy is not normally found in a hospital setting. However, the above-mentioned principles and method of non-directive play therapy can be implemented in the hospital setting with children who are suffering.

> In addition to the natural setting of school, several studies cited with children in hospital settings were conducted with children receiving other hospital services who might benefit from a play therapy treatment provided by hospital staff to reduce their anxiety.
>
> *Ray (2006, p. 147)*

Health play specialist

The role of a HPS plays a key part for children and their development. Jolly (1976, cited in Hubbuck 2009) states "The play specialist helps the child cope with the experience of being in hospital". This HPS still plays a key role after 50 years, where originally 'The Lady Greens' first interacted with children in hospital. In 1989 Save the Children Fund also recognised the importance of play (Figure 21.2).

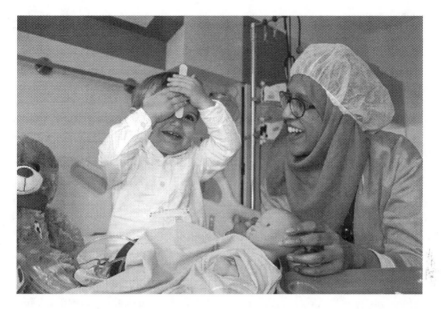

FIGURE 21.2   Rapport building session – inpatients room. (Picture taken by our marketing team with a child actor at Al Jalila Children Hospital)

CASE STUDY

As part of our service, the team worked closely with the oncology department, supporting the patients and their families. Services included the use of therapeutic play as a medium, and educational support to the patients' families during their time at the Children's Hospital, as inpatient and outpatient.

Here we introduce Zain (pseudonym), a six-year-old boy of Arab middle eastern heritage, diagnosed with T-Cell Acute Lymphoblastic Leukaemia. This was his first time in the hospital. The diagnosis was sudden and was a shock to the entire family. When he was first admitted to the Oncology Ward, Bushra (health play specialist) was contacted by the Head Nurse to assess and support him.

The provision of the play specialist – Bushra Ashraf

The patient was discussed at a multidisciplinary team (MDT) huddle and after hearing the handover my initial thoughts were to quickly meet the patient and his family. Before meeting Zain, there were some steps, which were important for the health play specialist to know. It was key to arrange a meeting with the relevant professionals to understand the history and background. Taberna et al. (2020) suggest the main purpose of an MDT is for different professionals to meet and put in place a treatment plan, which I have found to be most beneficial to get patient updates and adjust my approach accordingly.

After establishing the key information, I met Zain and introduced myself and my role. Rapport building was initiated to find out family dynamics; who were the main caregivers for Zain, and if there were things that may affect the admission, such as the new and strange environment, past medical experiences, and new unfamiliar people.

Building a rapport with Zain was crucial. He appeared calm and quiet. Normalising the situation through play was a great way to find out his likes and dislikes. The first month was very hard for Zain and there was a lot of silent treatment and moments of being mute. As professionals, we tried to find out the reasons behind this and daily visits to see Zain really helped to understand such issues. This young patient was missing his family life. For complex (and confidential) reasons the father was the main caregiver at the moment, and so he stayed with Zain for most of the day. This made Zain feel worse as he wanted to go home and was not able to understand the long admissions. Zain appeared depressed; this was becoming apparent to other staff members who also noticed the non-verbal behaviour. When we checked in with the nurses, they commented on his behaviour stating, "Zain talks to you but not us".

It took some time for Zain to feel safe around me as he was engaged in play through games, arts and crafts and many other fun and appealing activities, which enabled him to trust enough to talk to me. Zain participated in activities for the first two weeks after which he stopped talking and only responded in a baby voice. Regression during hospital admissions is something caused by stress (Youell, 2022). The new diagnosis was a traumatic event, which Zain was experiencing and may be a cause of his regression. After some time when revisiting Zain he did not want to engage in any play other than his tablet. I referred Zain to Gemma for play therapy and Sara for recreational therapy sessions to help him explore, understand, and work through his feelings. By making the referral it was a way for Zain to process his feelings and work through the regressive behaviour he was experiencing.

Most procedures were done in Zain's room as he was unable to leave due to his infection risk. Carrying out procedures in his room would normally be discouraged, because the room is his only safe place within the hospital, which could potentially raise his anxiety levels, which in turn could lead to a more traumatic experience, but unfortunately it was not possible to carry out procedures in a treatment room. Preparation for procedures such as a Portacath (port) insertion for example, and then accessing the port, was a key part of treatment and for the patient to understand why this had to be done. After the first preparation session, Zain was always keen to be shown what would happen and engaged well in medical play. Vakili et al. (2015) studied children who were prepared for surgery during hospital. One of the most important points identified was that when preparing children, it is important to seek clear and accurate information about the procedure. During medical play Zain was always keen to be shown his doll which had been made with the patient for accessing the port or being shown what was happening. This was also enabling a form of trust to be built with Zain and myself.

When working with Zain I shared a picture of a preparation doll for him to see (see Figures 21.3 and 21.4).

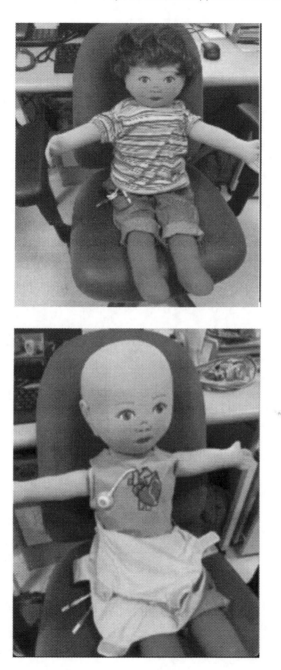

FIGURES 21.3 AND 21.4 Pictures of preparation dolls.

He chose to make his own, which he described as "mine". It was dressed in a hospital gown, with a name label. In the pictures shown to Zain, he was able to see where the port was and how it was accessed with the connectors. Of the two images one had hair, the other did not. This was a stage he would be faced with. My colleagues, Sara (the recreational therapist) and a psychologist, developed a therapeutic story for Zain, to help him process and accept his hair loss.

On daily ward rounds I was informed of any procedures Zain was having. This allowed me to prepare in advance and find resources to support him whilst having his port accessed or having general anaesthesia. Zain loved to play 'I spy' where we looked for things on the journey down to theatre. During pre-anaesthesia we played with a squishy ball to help calm Zain and I helped him focus on some breathing techniques. Zain's father was always present during this time and relied on me to be there early on theatre days. His father would comment "we were waiting for you; Zain really looks forward to playing games and seeing you". It was always emotional for Zain's father to see him go to theatre. After each procedure I spent time with his father and accompanied the nurse to reassure him that everything was ok. Sometimes his father would make a call to Zain's mother and update her on how well things had gone that morning.

Most healthcare professionals in the hospital do not see the importance of play and do not consider that children have heightened anxiety in a hospital setting. When supporting Zain for many of his procedures there were times of silence for him and his father. This was mainly based around being in hospital and facing heightened anxiety levels. There are different levels, for example, when he was newly diagnosed with his T Cell acute Lymphoblastic Leukaemia the anxiety was very severe, and his family was also affected.

Providing play interventions really supported Zain as he was able to be more relaxed, e.g. using breathing techniques and stress balls, and there were times when Zain asked for storybooks with 3D animations. Research by Fernandes et al. (2015) shows such methods help reduce anxiety levels for children who are hospitalised.

After surgery Zain would often be very hungry or sometimes not want to eat. He lost his appetite many times. As a health play specialist, it was also very important that such issues were addressed through play using positive reinforcement techniques, which did not always work with Zain. However, when Zain was well, he loved to eat; his favourite was chicken or Chinese food. During a one-to-one session he asked to have lunch with the Team, it was a good way to help Zain feel comfortable and it encouraged him to eat. By arranging the lunch date, Zain was given control as he was able to choose what he wanted to eat, and we could all eat this together.

Engaging Zain in play was very important. This mainly took place in his room, as he was not able to leave. However, there were times when Zain was given an exception. The playroom had to be blocked off for individual play sessions, allowing Zain to feel safe and express himself openly and feel at ease, so the playroom became a place of safety. Weinberger et al. (2017) describe this as a refuge. Zain's passion for play with cars was noted, and he could spend hours talking about each car and what he loves. This tool worked well when we were in the room as we would look out of the window and Zain would call out each car name in the car park, knowing which staff member had what car. When his father stayed Zain was also able to direct me to the family car. He was at his happiest moments during these times of play. Crenshaw and Kelly explain the importance of the hospital playroom thus: "to give children and their families a moment of spontaneous, non-demanding, untethered joy" (2018, p. 61).

Long-term patients like Zain celebrate many key parts of their life in hospital. In this case Zain celebrated his birthday, which was very important. As a play specialist it is my duty to make his time in hospital a positive experience; therefore, it was essential to arrange a birthday party for Zain. Zain made a list of people he wanted to invite; the theme was based around cars. Decorations were placed in the room ready for the celebration, and with Zain being unable to go home, the special occasion was marked on the ward. The staff sang happy birthday to Zain, and he was given presents.

As a health play specialist I was able to support Zain through this difficult time, while helping to prepare him for procedures, alongside providing advice and support for his family and a normalised environment in an unfamiliar and scary place.

The provision of play therapy – Gemma Hookins

A referral for play therapy was made by Bushra for Zain, a newly diagnosed admission to the Oncology Ward. Part of my initial assessment was to find out how he was feeling, showing understanding and then reflecting his thoughts and feelings back to him and helping him to feel heard and validated. I also explained to Zain who I was and that I would come and see him while he is in hospital and that we could play together. Furthermore, I asked questions to find out more about him, what he liked and disliked, and assessed his social and emotional development level. For the first part of his treatment and inpatient admission, he was bed-bound due to a high risk of infection. Therefore, most of the early play therapy sessions were in the ward-room. I explained to Zain the toys I had available, which he could then choose what he would like for me to bring for each session. For example, the expressive and creative arts, such as drawing, painting, clay, playdough, puppets, the sand tray with miniature figures, and Lego. These toys and materials could be easily moved around the hospital in a portable playtime bag (Figures 21.5 and 21.6).

All Parents completed the Goodman (1997) Strengths and Difficulties Questionnaire (SDQ), a tool that play therapists use as a baseline for qualitative evidence-based tracking of the effectiveness of the intervention. Furthermore, a parent questionnaire was used to gather information on the family and their main concerns and any additional stressors that needed to be taken into consideration.

In the first session I explained to Zain that he could choose what he would like to do; he chose the sand tray. I further explained that he could choose any

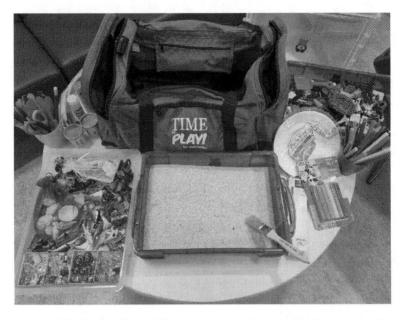

FIGURE 21.5 The hospital's portable resources, used to provide therapeutic play sessions in the medical wards. These toys and materials could be easily moved around the hospital in a portable playtime bag.

of the 'miniature' items to help him explore his feelings during this current situation, and if he liked he could tell his own story. Zain buried all the jewels, used the miniature figures such as angels and coffins, and symbolically explored death. He did this in silence, seeming to go deep into the subconscious world. In further sessions, he shifted from the sand tray to the expressive and creative

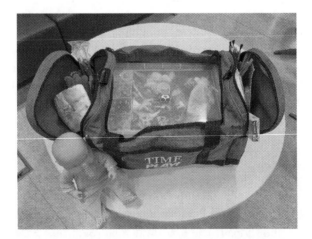

FIGURE 21.6 Play therapy portable sand and creative arts bag.

arts. He made 'friends' out of paper plates, which possibly symbolised his feelings around missing his friends and family while he felt 'stuck' within the hospital, as he would often speak about his baby brother.

Zain went through many processes throughout his time in the hospital, at the beginning he was open to exploration, and could verbalise his thoughts, and say what he didn't like about his treatment. However, through the middle stage, when he had been admitted for a very long period, and his nausea was daily, he withdrew. He stopped talking and regressed; he didn't laugh and didn't want to interact with anyone. However, during this stage, Zain allowed and still tolerated the play therapy sessions which was encouraging. He chose to use the sand tray during this difficult time, including the miniature figures. The sand tray became a bridge between the two worlds of phantasy and reality (Lowenfeld, 1993), bringing the unconscious to the conscious to gain mastery over it. He would work in silence processing his thoughts and feelings. He spent weeks continuing the same theme of burying objects; food items, treasure, family members, and leaving them buried. During this time, I reflected on his actions, which Axline (1974) suggests validates the child's experience and feelings.

After a few months of not speaking, a turning point came in play therapy, when he found the cars. He loved cars. He initiated a car race with me on the bedside table, a breakthrough! We raced the cars and we both let them fly off the end of the table. Zain looked at me and laughed. This was the first time in a long time that he really smiled; he had found joy again. From this point on the sand trays became more positive. He told his sand world stories of himself and his family on the farm with animals, swimming in the pool, which he seemed to enjoy. He was speaking about the future and seemed to accept his condition and was fighting back. Zain then continued to build his self-confidence and aided his self-regulation through setting challenges for himself with the Lego. In each session he made different objects, mainly animals and cars.

Once Zain was discharged from the hospital and returned for outpatient follow-up visits, I would see him in the hospital playroom to support him as he continued to build coping skills and self-confidence through his journey. Non-directive play therapy gave Zain the freedom to do what he needed to do for healing, working through difficult feelings and processing them, and finally mastering them. It also provided an environment in which he felt safe to be expressive, with an attuned play therapist who validated his thoughts and feelings, and gave him the time and opportunity to work through the difficult feelings that came during his hospital stay and subsequent treatments.

Reflection

Upon reflection, we can see Zain's journey from shock to denial, rejection, regression, and coming out the other side to acceptance, coping, and finding joy again. Zain was followed throughout his journey as an inpatient and outpatient, where we provided therapeutic support and continuity of care, for him and his family. Bushra provided a normalised environment and activities, further, preparing him for procedures, accompanying him to the operating theatre, providing distraction pre- and post-lumber punctures which reduced his anxiety. Gemma provided the opportunity for Zain to explore his feelings safely, using the creative and expressive arts, validating his experiences, and allowing for freedom of expression for Zain to process what was happening to him, so that he could gain mastery over it and find peace. Sara used directive and non-directive therapeutic interventions that helped Zain improve his quality of life, emotional support and coping, and overall functioning. Although we all use play as a medium and connection with our patients, each speciality has different approaches and outcomes.

In summary

The Child Life Team faced many challenges in setting up their play specialities. At first, the healthcare professionals did not understand and devalued our practices, and further, parents were wary of our service and thought we were only there to entertain or educate as teachers. However, when given proper resources explaining our practices, parents quickly understood and welcomed the interventions we offered. With dedication, education, and awareness it has been possible to establish this much needed service in our hospital setting where it has eventually been embraced and appreciated.

References

Axline, V.M. (1966) *Dibs, In search of Self.* London: Victor Gollancz

Axline, V.M. (1974) *Play Therapy.* New York, NY: Ballantine

Coyne, I. (2006) Children's experiences of hospitalization. *Journal of Child Health Care,* 10 (4) pp. 326–336

Crenshaw, D., & Kelly, J. (2018) Play Therapy in Assisting Children with Medical Challenges. In: Rubin, L. (ed.) *Handbook of Medical Play Therapy and Child Life.* New York, NY: Routledge

Else, P. (2012) *The Value of Play.* London: Continuum

Fernandes, S., Arriaga, P., & Esteves, F. (2015) Using an educational multimedia application to prepare children for outpatient surgeries. *Health Communication,* 30 (12) pp. 1190–1200

Goodman, R. (1997) *The Strengths and Difficulties Questionnaire: A Research Note.* [Online] Available from: <https://pubmed.ncbi.nlm.nih.gov/9255702/> [Accessed 10 December 2022]

Hubbuck, C. (2009) *Play for Sick Children: Play Specialists in Hospital and Beyond.* London: Jessica Kingsley Publishers

Jolly (1976) Why Children Must Be Able to Play in Hospital. *The Times,* 21 April 1976, cited in Hubbuck, C. (2009) *Play for Sick Children: Play Specialists in Hospital and Beyond.* London: Jessica Kingsley Publishers

Landreth, G. (2012) *Play Therapy: The Art of Relationship,* Third Edition. New York, NY: Routledge

Lowenfeld, M. (1993) *Understanding Children's Sandplay: Lowenfeld's World Technique*. London: The Margaret Lowenfeld Trust

Prasetya, F. (2021) The Effect of Colouring Pictures Treatment on Anxiety in Pre-school Age Patient Hospitalized at Baladhika Husada Hospital Jember. In: Proceedings of the 4th International AgroNursing Conference, 'Optimizing The Role of Nursing and Health Professionals to Enhance Health Care Quality in The New Normal Era.' [Online] e-Proceeding, [S.l.], pp. 43–47, Sep. 2021. ISSN 2686-0783. Available from: <https://jurnal.unej.ac.id/index.php/prosiding/article/view/26681> [Accessed 19 June 2022]

Ray, D. (2006) Evidence-Based Play Therapy. In: Schaefer, E. & Kaduson, H. (eds) *Contemporary Play Therapy: Theory, Research, and Practice*. New York, NY: The Guildford Press

Rogers, C. (1942) *Counselling and Psychotherapy*. Boston, MA: Houghton Mifflin Company

Rogers, C. (1951) *Client-centred Therapy: It's Current Practice Implications and Theory*. Boston, MA: Houghton Mifflin Company

Save the Children Fund (1989) *Hospital: A Deprived Environment for Children? The Case for Hospital Playschemes*. London: Save the Children

Taberna, M., Moncayo, F., Salas, E., Antonio, M., Arribas, L., Vilajosana, E., Torres, E. & Mesia, R. (2020) The multidisciplinary team (MDT) approach and quality of care. *Frontiers of Oncology*, 10 (85) [Online] Available from: <https://www.ncbi.nlm.nih.gov/pmc/articles/PMC7100151/> [Accessed 19 June 2022]

Vakili, R., Abbasi, M., Hashemi, A., Khademi, G. & Saedi, M. (2015) Preparing a child for surgery and hospitalization. *International Pediatrics*, 3 (3.1) pp. 599–605

Weinberger, N., Butler, A., McGee, B., Schumacher, P. & Brown R. (2017) Child life specialists' evaluation of hospital playroom design: A mixed method inquiry. *Journal of Interior Design*, 42 (2) pp. 71–91

Yateem, N., Brenner, M., Shorrab, A. & Docherty, C. (2016) Play distraction versus pharmacological treatment to reduce anxiety levels in children undergoing day surgery: A randomized controlled non-inferiority trial. *Child: Care, Health and Development*, 42 (4) pp. 572–581

Youell, J. (2022) *Understanding Regression Psychology*. Better Help [Online] Available from: < https://www.betterhelp.com/advice/psychologists/understanding-regression-psychology/> [Accessed 19 June 2022]

22

"G'DAY!"

A history of hospital play in an Australian children's hospital

Leanne Hallowell – Previously Head of Educational Play Therapy, Royal Children's Hospital, Melbourne

Play in hospital is not a new concept. Play in hospital does not happen by chance.

Play in hospital can be found in a variety of wards, departments and specialist areas.

Play in hospital occurs in many countries throughout the world.

Hospital play services are valuable in supporting children and their families during hospital admissions and medical care. However, these play services can look quite different in varying settings. Similarly, the title given to those who work to provide play in hospitals varies from one country to the next. The prioritisation of play in hospital varies as does the types of play which is engaged in. Often these differences have come about as a response to widely varied social attitudes and political structures.

Recognising these differences, this chapter provides a background to the development of the hospital play service in one specific Australian hospital, the Royal Children's Hospital in Melbourne:

> *The author acknowledges that this chapter was written whilst on the traditional lands of the Wurundjeri people of the Kulin nation, and pays respect to Elders both past, present and emerging. The Royal Children's Hospital, referred to in these pages, was built on Wurundjeri land.*

Introduction

In 1870, 35 years after white settlement occurred on the land of the Wurundjeri peoples, the population of Melbourne was around 200,000 people. It should be noted that indigenous populations were not counted in census data at that time.

Discoveries of gold in the 1850s meant that Melbourne became a fast growing and wealthy city. That wealth was unequal, and Melbourne became a city of

DOI: 10.4324/9781003255444-27

contrasts. Whilst some areas were tree lined streets with large expansive mansions, pockets of the township were slums. The unequal distribution of wealth meant those who were destitute became more so. Infrastructure development could not keep up with the rapid growth resulting in poor housing, inadequate supply of water, unhygienic disposal of sewerage and displaced families. Women were often deserted and left with children, whilst the fathers headed to the gold fields.

The slums were areas of significant poverty, with poor sanitation. Widespread inadequate nutrition resulted in malnutrition rendering children susceptible to diseases including "diphtheria, tuberculosis of the hip – 'the hip disease' – or the big killer, the 'Typhoid Fiend'" (Murdoch 1991, p. xi) as were whooping cough, scarlet fever, tuberculosis, measles, dysentery, diarrhoea, bronchitis and pneumonia. The mortality rate of children under five years of age was reported at 34% (Singleton, 1870).

Hospitals are established to heal the sick. The sickest people are found in areas where rates of poverty and destitution are significant. Accordingly, the Hospital for Sick Children in Melbourne opened in 1870 near to these slums (CDH 1877) and treated children as outpatients until the committee was able to buy six beds in December 1870 (Yule, 1999).

Philanthropy and the power of women

Children who live in poor conditions or with ill health stir natural sympathy. The society of Melbourne saw the need for a hospital for sick children and gave their philanthropy that has been fostered and maintained since foundation. Hospitals at this time, known as charity hospitals, were for those who could not afford doctors' fees. The funding of hospitals themselves came mainly from donations.

It was women who formed the first committee of the Hospital for Sick Children. Women with significant social influence, and ties to rich and powerful individuals within the colony, were recognised as 'energetic advocates' (HSC, 1876). This committee was not part of the written constitution, however their connections gave them considerable power, as did their strengths, determination and abilities. In selecting new members, careful consideration was given to what new members could provide for the hospital. The committee controlled every aspect of how the hospital was run, from policy decisions related to finance and buildings, to details of nursing rosters and children's meals. The committee was not concerned with medical treatments, although they did take an interest in the general welfare of individual patients.

The early history of the hospital shows that the focus was one of caring for ill children, with limited resources, including staff. Doctors were mainly honorary, and paediatrics was not a recognised specialty. The hospital itself was committed to providing a space for sick children to go to be cared for. As successful as the committee was at raising money and applying for government grants, all funds raised were given over to covering day-to-day running costs. Any monies required for capital works required the committee to organise sponsored events.

Given the social and political context of the time we could assume that the psychological and sociological needs of the children were not well considered. However, in early records of the hospital it is noted that the women of the committee were concerned about the children, concerned that they received good food, and refusing to allow nurses to punish children by 'withholding their pudding' (Yule, 1999). It was also noted that there was a shortage of toys for the children to play with. Nurses were under instruction to keep the children happy and amused and disciplinary action was harsh for those nurses who, on rare occasions, were found being unkind to any of the children (Yule, 1999).

The role of medical staff in developing play in hospital

Historian Peter Yule wrote in the *The Royal Children's Hospital: A History of Faith, Science and Love* (1999), that whilst the committee and wider community, saw a need for a children's hospital, the specific reasons for its existence still needed to be made explicit, in particular within the medical profession. Arguments supporting a specialised hospital for children, found in the first annual report, included:

- The 'moral evil' that resulted from the association of children with adults in general hospitals
- Specific needs of children in relation to nursing, diet and fresh air
- Hospitals for children had successfully been established in Britain and Europe
- Half of all deaths in Victoria were of children under the age of five years

AMJ (1887)

The last of these points is perhaps the most striking.

The second annual report in 1888 made a further point that the sights and sounds in general hospitals are not adapted to the needs of children, and "too often leave impressions that can never be effaced" (Yule, 1999, p. 17).

By the turn of the century and beyond, the place of play within children's care begins to emerge in the records of the time. A kindergarten was established in the 1920s, the Annie Stirling Kindergarten. The focus was to provide play for ambulant patients but by the 1930s, doctors, such as Dr Douglas Galbraith and Dr Stanley Williams, were asking for provision to be made for entertainment and amusement for long term ward patients. In the orthopaedic section, Dr Galbraith referred to "treating children as children and not as disabled children" (Yule, 1999, p. 214). Similarly, in 1935 the medical superintendent Dr Stanley Williams, requested for provision to be made for 'entertainment and amusement' of the patients in the Venereal Diseases (VD) Ward', since these children were in hospital for lengthy periods and it was considered that it would be "of distinct advantage if their minds could be occupied in the direction indicated" (Yule, 1999, p. 262). Dr Galbraith was quite successful, and entertainment and activities were provided in the orthopaedic section; Dr Williams less so, as staff from the kindergarten refused to work on the VD ward.

In the planning of the new hospital, which opened in 1962, Dr Vernon Collins (medical superintendent) ensured that playrooms were part of each ward. He had seen playrooms whilst working in the United Kingdom. Although planned, there was no ward-based play staff until the mid-1970s. Until then, playrooms were often used for storage.

The role of nurses in developing play in hospital

Nurses were expected to provide play experiences for children in the early days of the hospital. Grace Jennings Carmichael (1991), a nurse at the Hospital for Sick Children, wrote of beds being moved to the windows so that the children could see the pupils at the nearby schools playing in the school grounds (p. 32). Carmichael recounted providing toys for bed bound children (p. 81) – ensuring they were removed from the bed before the doctor arrived! – and of how much music was enjoyed by all children. This was provided by a musical-box, accompanied by the children themselves on mouth organs or whistles, or by violinists who would come to the hospital to play (pp. 81–82). Further, Carmichael wrote that the wards were not a "dreary expanse of white suffering faces" but rather were full of "rowdy boisterous natures that would convert the ward into a football ground" after a doctor encouraged "a spirited round of playing catches, during which the balls fly around the beds amid a chorus of boy voices that never seem to belong to sick children" (p. 31).

Nurses continued to play with children in a variety of ways, although it began to be noted that, like the doctors, they increasingly became more focused on treating disease and the non-medical needs of children were at times neglected. Play was noted as an effective distraction by nurses in the 1950s. Yule (1999) describes how a nurse was seen to turn a child away from a bedside ward round, as the child made it known that he was not happy with the process. The nurse then distracted the child with some toys. The ward round was being conducted by Dr Howard Williams, the medical superintendent, who then explained to the round the importance of supporting children according to their developmental age.

In a doctoral thesis undertaken by Dr Judi Parson (2009), it was noted that nurses continued to engage in forms of play with children. However, it was often based on need to get through a procedure or treatment, rather than for the developmental or psychosocial needs of the child.

Rehabilitation and play

In the 1920s and 1930s children with infantile paralysis, osteomyelitis, tubercular hip and polio were sent to the separate orthopaedic section of the Hospital for Sick Children, which was 54 miles from the main hospital in

Melbourne. Visiting hours were for just two hours on Sundays. Many children did not have visitors due to distance to and lack of ability to travel by family members.

Over 80% of the children admitted to the orthopaedic section of the Hospital for Sick Children were hospitalised for over a year due to their specific condition. The staff, recognising that treatment alone was not enough for this cohort of children, developed a philosophy which noted that their social, educational and vocational needs were to be considered. A school was established on site, by the Education Department to support children's learning from kindergarten (five years old) to merit certificate (14 years old). Further occupational therapy was instigated to support children to develop skills which would be helpful in obtaining employment. In further attempts to support children living in the orthopaedic section, activities made available to the children included Boy Scouts and Girl Guides, and a craft hostel. Regular movie nights were held, and the children were visited by entertainers and sportsmen. Birthdays were celebrated as they were considered by Dr Galbraith, the medical superintendent of the unit, to be especially important for children who were long stay patients (Yule, 1999).

Social contexts of medical care were changing at this time. Medical, Nursing and Allied Health Professionals recognised not only the need to keep children occupied but also the need to provide education and skills for a life beyond the hospital. It was thought that by providing a level of education and occupational skills, children would not be a cost to the community in the form of becoming 'invalid pensioners' (as reported in The Herald, July, 1934, cited in Yule, 1999, p. 215), but would be active contributing members of the community.

Schools in hospital

The hospital received Royal Assent in 1953, after seven years of lobbying by the committee. It was 1969 before a school was established at the main campus of the Royal Children's Hospital, annexed to the school at the orthopaedic section. The space was leased in the hospital and the staff employed by the Education Department. The focus was to maintain normal schooling, be that in the classroom or at a child's bedside.

Tensions did occur between the school and the 'Educational Play Therapists', as they had become known. These difficulties were largely around how to delineate which children were referred to which department and for what reasons. With some playrooms being open to all, there was a drifting of children into the playrooms, regardless of school timetable requirements. The hospital kindergarten had stopped operating in 1959, and the existing play staff at that time were not able to have a presence on every ward. There was a gap in service provision.

Kindergarten and play

The Annie Stirling Kindergarten ran at the hospital from 1926 to 1959. The committee of the kindergarten and the kindergarten itself became an auxiliary of the Occupational Therapy Department in 1959. Children who were able to leave the ward could go to the occupational therapy playroom each morning for play and craft activities. However, Occupational Therapists were unhappy at being seen and referred to as 'play ladies'.

In the mid-1970s there was a convergence of activities and provision of play. Discussions commenced which included nurses and allied health professionals, about the lack of staff, money and equipment to provide adequate play opportunities for ward-based children. Changes to clinical practices and treatments meant that fewer children could leave the wards. Some treatments and conditions resulted in more children being in isolation rooms. The need for play was now more apparent and discussions turned to asking what play could be provided on the wards and in those empty ward-based playrooms.

Play on the wards

Discussions about the non-medical needs of the children piqued the interest of Dr Alan Williams and his wife Dorothy Williams (previously a kindergarten teacher) who had observed the play programme at Great Ormond Street Hospital in London in 1977. Around the same time, another paediatrician, Dr Ian Stewart, carried out a research project entitled *How Children Spend Their Time in the Wards* (noted in Yule, 1999, p. 537). In 1977, with the support of the Occupational Therapy Department, a position for a play specialist was made available and Fiona Anderson was recruited from Great Ormond Street to start a play programme in Melbourne. This was a success, and with the support of nursing and medical staff, the hospital administration decided to expand the programme with the appointment of 12 play specialists.

The growth of the play department took a step backwards when two crises occurred. The resignation of a department head saw the department returned to Occupational Therapy Department until a new play department head could be found. State government funding was removed as a 'cost cutting measure' by a recently elected state government.

To some extent the latter was a benefit. Hospital Administration, under the direction of the then Chief Executive Officer, Ivor Davies, was able to fund some play positions under hospital recurrent funding. Educational Play Therapy was then able to stand alone from 1990 and had direct line reports, funding and management, into the hospital itself. Regardless, this was not enough to fund and cover all requests for educational play therapists. This author recollects that on her starting in the position as Head of Department in 1993, that within a week, she had been contacted by all Nurse Unit Managers to meet – each meeting was either about not reducing hours of play staff for their wards or to ask for a service or additional services.

Developing specialised play and working with others

Play staff started to engage more with children in need of more specialised play including diversion, distraction, hospital medical play and procedural pain management. As these specialised play services have developed at the Royal Children's Hospital in Melbourne, play staff on wards have gradually been recognised for their contributions to the psychosocial well-being of children. Key to this development were connections made in between practitioners at the hospital and a willingness to find ways to collaborate and respond to the needs of children and their families. Many of the following projects started simply as conversations in corridors or at staff functions – and then a willingness to try something different.

- The Practice MRI project: A lead MRI technologist wondered if play staff could help by supporting children to understand and manage the requirements of MRI scans, thereby reducing the need for a general anaesthetic (GA). A small project was set up. The success of the project resulted in a significant reduction in GA needs, and in getting more children through the hospital's waiting lists (Hallowell et al., 2008; de Amorim e Silva et al., 2006). This project also resulted in two masters degrees by play staff, a series of papers (see reference list), and awards from the Victorian State Government and the journal Pediatric Radiology. Further, this project was cost neutral. Children and their families were mainly seen as outpatients. The funding arrangements in Victoria, at the time, were that the hospital was paid for every outpatient appointment carried out – and this covered the salary of play staff working in that area and any resources they used. Further the need for anaesthetists, anaesthetics and recovery nurses was reduced. Other areas of the radiology department requested more play support and additional play staff were appointed to work only within Radiology.
- Funding was made available to the Educational Play Therapy Department and the Educational Resource Centre to re-establish an in-house television programme that could be broadcast to children when they were inpatients. 'Going Nuts with Macadamia' (now known as Be Positive) provided a space for departments to talk to children about what they did and also became integral to fund raising (RCH TV, 2022).
- As the hospital's Educational Play Therapists became known for their work in non-pharmacological pain management, they were asked to be involved in the establishment of Comfort Kids, a pain management programme, and were recognised as leading trainers for other hospital staff in the area (RCH, 2022).
- Connections to and involvement with national and international professional bodies representing hospital play services – namely the Australian Association of Hospital Play Specialists, Hospital Play Specialists Association of Aotearoa New Zealand, National Association of Hospital Play Specialists

(NAHPS) and the Association of Child Life Professionals (ACLP). These networks have provided spaces to connect via hospital visits and conference attendance to share and develop knowledge.

Across Australia, the role of play specialists has had different trajectories, depending on the State and the specific hospitals and departments that play staff work in. It is the reason the name, the definition of the work, the establishment of departments (or working within other departments), qualifications and funding have varied. The establishment of the national Australasian Association of Hospital Play Specialists in 1984 helped the recognition of these. The organisation underwent a rebranding in 2014 to become the Association of Child Life Therapists Australia (ACLTA, 2014).

Conclusion

This appears to be a brief history of play in one Australian hospital, and in many ways it is. It also highlights some important factors relating to how play as a discipline can become embedded within healthcare organisations. It is still the case that not all hospitals in Australia, even those where there are paediatric patients, have play as part of the support for children and their families. For those hospitals who do have established play services, mainly large paediatric hospitals, the way it has developed has been based on a variety of factors.

Funding was and still is crucial. Each state in Australia has a slightly different funding model, which needs to be navigated. Funding at The Royal Children's Hospital in Melbourne was only made available for the Educational Play Therapy Department through recurrent hospital funds, when funds provided by state government departments not connected to health were withdrawn. Recognised as a stand-alone department, and with the development of technology and advancements in health care, there has been a shift in focus from familiar 'normalising' play, which is a key part of healthy childhood (Hubbuck, 2009), to include using play as a tool to support children requiring healthcare including but not limited to distraction, coping and medical preparation. Discipline heads within an independent department have autonomy to focus on the work of the discipline itself and support staff via targeted professional development, with funds less likely to be shifted to other areas. Further they can manage staff to best suit current needs and requirements of the patients and their treatment.

Play, as an independent department, has also been very successful at attracting funding, as a single entity or in conjunction with other departments. A willingness to engage and 'tell our stories' to philanthropic groups keeps a focus on play and also keeps money coming in. Stories are told at local levels, from school groups, and charitable groups, such as craft groups (where a lot of play resource, including blank body outline dolls are donated from), to larger corporations who have provided funds for larger programmes. These stories were added to and retold, developing relationships between the play department and the funding body and shifting one-off donations to ongoing funding relationships.

At the RCH the connections made with medical, nursing and allied health staff have been key to the development of the play service. It was by being able to work with these other professions, as part of multidisciplinary teams that allowed for projects to be developed and for the work to meet the specific needs of the children and families in attendance. It also meant there were opportunities for research, joint publications and conference presentations. Increasing the visibility, by any means available, has made Educational Play Therapy known and recognised as a department within Allied Health.

Regardless of the political and social context, those engaged in play in hospitals need to find ways to understand and make a case for play provision and, by doing so, to support children and their families in their medical journey. The history of play at The Royal Children's Hospital in Melbourne indicates how understanding the complexity of funding, and the development of connections to those with power within the organisations in which we work, is vital.

References

ACLTA (2014) *Hospital Play and Child Life Therapy in Australia: A Short History* Association of Child Life Therapists Australia. [Online] Available from: <http://childlife.org.au/documents/history-chart.html> [Accessed 31 July2022].

AMJ (1887) First Annual Report. Hospital for Sick Children, in Australian Medical Journal, 1887, cited in Yule (1999). *The Royal Children's Hospital. A History of Faith, Science and Love.* Rushcutters Bay, NSW: Halstead.

Carmichael, G.J. (1991) *Hospital Children: Sketches of Life and Character in the Childrens Hospital, Melbourne.* Main Ridge, Victoria: Loch Haven Books. (originally published in 1891 by G. Robertson)

CDH (1877) A Contagious Diseases Hospital. *Australian Medical Journal* (January 1877), pp. 10–11. [Online] Available from: <https://rest.neptune-prod.its.unimelb.edu.au/server/api/core/bitstreams/4163467f-ed57-5346-9f4a-844663f672e5/content> [Accessed 31 July 2022].

de Amorim e Silva, C., Mackenzie, A., Hallowell, L., Stewart, S. & Ditchfield, M. (2006). Practice MRI: Reducing the Need for Sedation and General Anaesthesia in Children Undergoing MRI. *Australasian Radiology* 50, pp. 319–323.

Hallowell, L., Stewart, S., de Amorim e Silva, C. & Ditchfield, M. (2008). Reviewing the Process of Preparing Children for MRI. *Pediatric Radiology* 38 (3), pp. 271–279.

HSC (1876) The Hospital for Sick Children. *Australian Medical Journal* (August 1876) pp. 267–268. [Online] Available from: <https://rest.neptune-prod.its.unimelb.edu.au/server/api/core/bitstreams/da5f507f-4ab0-5862-b7d8-5da268a8c9c6/content> [Accessed 31 July 2022].

Hubbuck, C. (2009) *Play for Sick Children. Play Specialists in Hospitals and Beyond.* London: Jessica Kingsley Publishers.

Murdoch, E. (1991) Introduction to the 100th Anniversary Edition of Carmichael, G. (1891) *Hospital Children. Sketches and Character in the Children's Hospital, Melbourne.* Main Ridge, Vic: Loch Haven Books. (Original work published by George Robertson & Co.)

Parson J. (2009) *Integration of procedural play for children undergoing cystic fibrosis treatment: A nursing perspective* [PhD Thesis]. Central Queensland University: Brisbane.

RCH (2022) About Comfort Kids. [Online] Available from: <https://www.rch.org.au/comfortkids/> [Accessed 31 July 2022].

RCH TV (2022) *RCH TV Be Positive (B+)*. [Online] Available from: https://www.rch.org.au/be-positive/> [Accessed 31 July 2022].

Singleton, J. (1870) On the Mortality of Victoria. *Australian Medical Journal* (December 1870), pp. 365–368. [Online] Available from: <https://rest.neptune-prod.its.unimelb.edu.au/server/api/core/bitstreams/89d01266-4c94-5705-b91a-548861884f1a/content> [Accessed 29 July 2022].

Yule, P. (1999) *The Royal Children's Hospital. A History of Faith, Science and Love*. Rushcutters Bay, NSW: Halstead Press.

23

INTEGRATING PLAY IN NORTH AMERICAN HOSPITALS

Historical and current approaches

Michael Patte – Program Coordinator: Child Life Specialist and Playwork Certificate/Minor Programs

Emma Plank is considered the 'founding mother' of the Child Life movement in America. Due in part to her seminal book, *Working with Children in Hospitals* (1962), she is widely credited with bringing play into the hospital setting. In 1955 Plank was invited by the Nobel Laureate, Dr Fred Robbins, to create a programme to address the social, emotional, and educational needs of hospitalised children at the Cleveland City Children's Hospital. Plank highlighted that hospital settings were not child friendly environments and that prolonged separation from primary caregivers during hospitalisation had negative physical and psychological effects, a condition known as hospitalism (Spitz, 1945). Although she accepted that children's nurses were inherently compassionate people, Plank found being compassionate does not necessarily mean you see the full context of your workplace clearly. In reality, children's wards were not at all child-centred.

I had my own experience of hospitalism in the 1970s when (as a child) I developed pneumonia and spent several days in isolation in an oxygen tent, with no one able to ease my fears. My mother was not allowed to spend the night with me in the hospital. Perhaps that is why I became interested in play within the hospital setting when attending the 2006 conference of the Association for the Study of Play (TASP). At that conference, I attended Fraser Brown's presentation about working with abandoned children in a Romanian children's hospital. I also attended a seminar by one of the founders of the modern child life profession, Rosemary Bolig (1984) where she summarised the five central themes of the child life field: (a) diversion, (b) activity, (c) therapeutic, (d) child development, and (e) comprehensive. As a direct result of these two inspirational presentations and many years of hard work, I developed two minor programmes at Bloomsburg University with play at their core, i.e. child life specialist and playwork (Patte, 2020).

DOI: 10.4324/9781003255444-28

According to the American Academy of Pediatrics:

> Child life specialists focus on the optimal development and wellbeing of infants, children, adolescents, and young adults while promoting coping skills and minimizing the adverse effects of hospitalization, health care, and/or other potentially stressful experiences. Using therapeutic play, expressive modalities, and psychological preparation as primary tools, in collaboration with the entire health care team and family, child life interventions facilitate coping and adjustment at times and under circumstances that might prove overwhelming for the child.
>
> *American Academy of Pediatrics (2014)*

Emma Plank's work served as the impetus for the development of the child life profession, initially in the form of several independent organisations which eventually came together as the Association of Child Life Professionals (ACLP). The ACLP is now the certifying body for all child life professionals in North America. In order to obtain certification, candidates must possess a Bachelor's Degree that contains ten required ACLP courses and also successfully complete a 600-hour clinical internship under the supervision of a certified child life specialist (CCLS).

There are now around 400 children's hospitals across the USA, Canada, and Mexico, and the field of child life can now be found in countries around the world including Australia, Japan, and Kuwait (Fein et al., 2012; Hicks, 2008). The number of child life specialists in any setting varies according to the size of the hospital, and they often develop a close link with specialist areas (intensive care, paediatric sedation, birth to 12 years, and various in-patient wards). The work is sometimes age-related, and the child life specialism is practised in many other venues (paediatric dentists, funeral homes, palliative care, therapeutic camps, etc.).

The child life programme aims to help children transition between environments – firstly from home to hospital and eventually from hospital back into the outside world. It begins with an assessment of their point on the developmental continuum to enable the team to provide appropriate help. This feeds into the preparation for medical procedures and helps with post-procedural mastery. Everything is geared to helping the child survive in this unnatural environment. There is great stress on the fact that this is a very unusual environment, and the child should still be able to play, i.e. continue one of the most 'normal' activities of life. Burns-Nader and Hernandez-Reif (2016) suggest that the programme emphasises three common types of play:

- Normative – nuanced by the child's status in hospital
- Medical – often messy and making use of hospital equipment, e.g. syringe art
- Therapeutic – promoting coping skills and psycho-social well-being, e.g. using puppets

In 2014 the Child Life Council (now ACLP) reported on their survey of current play practice in North America. The research was funded by the Walt Disney Foundation and found:

- One hundred per cent of children's hospitals had multiple playrooms, but with a variety of opening hours. Most were staffed by child life specialists and volunteers.
- Some playrooms were unstaffed.
- Forty per cent had some outdoor space, usually with play structures – mostly staffed.
- Various types of play were offered – either in playrooms, procedural rooms, or at the bedside.
- The most popular play types were crafts (97%), construction (96)%, games, expressive art, child-centred medical play (88%), dramatic (77%), gross motor play (76%), and loose parts (70%).
- Some hospitals also had pet therapy, special events, gurney-journeys, etc.
- The play type most used by child life specialists was medical play (99%).

McCue (1988) suggests medical play activities can be divided into four conceptual categories:

1. Role rehearsal/role reversal play – children taking on the roles of health care providers and re-enacting medical procedures on dolls or puppets
2. Fantasy play – making use of loose parts or standard play materials that are not medical equipment, where the child is reluctant to engage with medical play materials
3. Indirect play – more structured and goal-oriented, aiming to help the child engage with the medical environment through hospital-themed play materials and games
4. Medical art – more process-oriented, encouraging the child to use art materials to express themselves in relation to their medical experiences

The Child Life Council (2014) also asked about the hospitals' formal written policies. There appeared to be no great consistency across the country, let alone within each hospital. Although 64% of Programme Directors identified children's play as important in a patient's recovery plan, only 39% had a play policy. While 98% of the respondents had a toy cleansing policy, somewhat ironically only 14% saw stringent infection control as an issue worthy of a policy. The other 86% do not seem to think about that. On the other hand, 28% had a policy regarding the presence of siblings in the playroom.

There is a similar disconnect when it comes to play training. Only 14% of Programme Directors thought new members of staff were adequately trained, but only 25% provided in-service training. Nevertheless, 64% of child life specialists said they provide play training for other members of staff, and as many as

84% of Programme Directors claimed they encourage play innovation, creativity, and imaginative play.

Finally, the Programme Directors were asked what they thought were the barriers to play in hospitals. Their responses were:

- Inadequate staffing – 45%
- Lack of time – 45%
- Lack of space – 35%
- Lack of understanding about the value of play – 18%
- Infection control regulations – 14%
- Isolation precautions – 14%
- Patient's personal factors, e.g. medical fragility – 6%

The Child Life Council's report (2014) made a number of suggestions regarding how these barriers might be overcome. Not surprisingly, in light of their findings, they recommended the development of hospital play policies. They also wished to tackle the thorny issue of training, and so they called for an expansion of professional training opportunities, coupled with a revision of their own competencies framework, to include higher quality standards regarding play. They recommended the organisation of additional play groups, as well as providing more space for play and improving patient access to that space. Alongside offering a greater variety of play opportunities, they recognized the generally poor quality of play materials in hospitals. Therefore, they recommended the securing of materials for play with high play values.

Having said all that, I feel obliged to present my personal experience to the current situation. Sadly, in my clinical experience less than 20% of the child life specialist's work is focused on normative play. That is despite the generally accepted fact that when hospital wards are more 'normalized', children do not need so many medications and generally recover faster. It is an unfortunate fact of life that, in order to justify their positions, child life specialists have to be seen as productive. In the hospital environment that inevitably means the elements of CCLS work that impact directly on the priorities of the medical team are the ones that move to the fore. Hence, preparation for medical procedures and distraction work often take up a disproportionate amount of the CCLS's time. It is also the case that for infection control reasons, playrooms tend to be stocked with a limited range of toys, and that also has an impact on the potential for 'normalized' play.

Here is a personal experience that illustrates the sometimes unnoticed value of the child life specialist – in particular the value of normalised play.

Today a patient accidentally dislodged his breathing tube, causing unplanned extubation to occur. The Pediatric Intensive Care Unit sprang into action, and I worked with the patient and his father to provide procedural and emotional

> support. Throughout the procedure I held the patient's hand, as he was agitated and physically uncomfortable. I stayed by the patient's side until the procedure was complete, and he was relaxed and comfortable.
>
> Later in the day, I stopped by to provide normative play for the patient in the form of a favourite board game and to offer information about the pet therapy programme in the hospital. As I left the room, the patient's father said he really appreciated the care I provided his son throughout the day and actually said that I had the most important job, which was to provide a sense of normalcy in the stressful medical setting. If you were to ask me at the time of the procedure whether the father even knew I was in the room, I would say probably not. He seemed distracted and distraught because his son was in pain. However, his comment holds an important lesson: no act of kindness, no matter how small or seemingly insignificant, ever goes unnoticed.
>
> *Patte (2010)*

The CLC report (2014) also made suggestions regarding the sort of research that might be beneficial to the current state of play in North American hospitals. This included investigating the benefits of loose parts play and the extent to which adult-led play was occurring at the expense of child-initiated play. They also suggested examining the impact of education, staffing, and supervision on opportunities for play in medical settings. The final recommendation was to undertake research into the way in which CCLSs train parents about the value of play.

Since its early days, play has been at the heart of the child life profession. Although volumes of research emphasise play's vital role in the psychosocial and muscular-skeletal development of children in medical settings, the CLC report (2014) and my own experience suggest its application throughout North American hospitals is mixed. Various societal and institutional barriers marginalising play appear to have increased in recent years. CCLS need to ensure that the widespread trivialisation of the value of play is not allowed to intrude into the hospital environment. After all, play embodies the very essence of our beautiful profession.

References

American Academy of Pediatrics (2014) Child life services: Committee on hospital care and Child Life Council. *Pediatrics*, Vol. 133: 5, pp. 1471–1478.

Bolig, R. (1984) *Play in Hospital Settings*. Abingdon: Routledge.

Burns-Nader, S. & Hernandez-Reif, M. (2016). Facilitating play for hospitalized children through child life services. *Children's Health Care*, Vol. 45: 1, pp. 1–21.

Child Life Council (2014) *Report on Findings of Play Practices and Innovations Survey: The State of Play in North American Hospitals*. Rockville, MD: Child Life Council.

Fein, J., Zempsky, W., & Cravero, J. (2012). Relief of pain and anxiety in pediatric patients in emergency medical systems. *Pediatrics*, Vol. 130: 5, pp. 1391–1405.

Hicks, M. (2008). *Child Life beyond the Hospital*. Rockville, MD: Child Life Council.

McCue, K. (1988). Medical play: An expanded perspective. *Children's Health Care*, Vol. 16: 3, pp. 75–85.

Patte, M. (2010) *Field Notes Taken during a Child Life Internship*. Unpublished.

Patte, M. (2020). What is the state of play? Playful professions. *International Journal of Play*, Vol. 9: 3, pp. 1–4.

Plank, E. (1962) *Working with Children in Hospitals*. London: Tavistock Publications.

Spitz, R. (1945) Hospitalism: An inquiry into the genesis of psychiatric conditions in early childhood. *Psychoanalytic Study of the Child*, Vol. 1, pp. 53–74.

Website

Association of Child Life Professionals (ACLP) – https://www.childlife.org/

24

THE HOSPITAL PLAY SPECIALIST EDUCATION COURSE IN JAPAN

What we have achieved and what we need to overcome

Chika Matsudaira – Associate Professor of the University of Shizuoka

Fifteen years ago, the education of Hospital Play Specialists (HPS) began in Japan. This education programme started at the Junior College of the University of Shizuoka – the institution to which the writer belongs – as a project commissioned by the Ministry of Education, Culture, Sports, Science and Technology. Since then, 214 HPSs have been educated with the principle that through hospital play, sick children will understand more about their medical condition and this will reduce their anxiety and fear undergoing treatment.

When the education programme started, the goals were:

- To bring childcare workers and nurses back into paediatric healthcare settings with new knowledge and skills.
- To re-educate staff and improve conditions in children's hospital and paediatric care.
- To establish the HPS training curriculum so that other universities can start running the same HPS programme.
- To provide a platform for professional development and support for professionals involved in paediatric care. Such support networks are still few in number.

After 15 years, the Japanese HPS education programme finds itself moving forward with a new purpose. We have found that in order to create an environment in which all children can access hospital play, it is necessary to inform people more widely about what play means to sick children. We have needed to show this to the other professionals within paediatric multidisciplinary teams (MDT). There have also been changes made to the way HPS training is funded. The funding was originally part of a government scheme to encourage professionals

DOI: 10.4324/9781003255444-29

who work with adults to undertake vocational retraining. We are now moving towards a more established programme for individuals who are already working in paediatric healthcare to undertake the training.

This chapter describes the social problems faced by children in Japan and the consideration required of HPSs working with sick children in Japanese hospitals in light of these issues.

Children of high risk in Japan

Before the COVID-19 pandemic, many foreigners visited Japan as tourists, enjoying the country's culture, food and hospitality. From the point of view of children's welfare, however, we see not a country of abundance, but a society that pushes children into a corner. Japan's child poverty rate is among the worst in the world's Organisation for Economic Co-operation and Development (OECD) countries. This has risen since the 1980s – the child poverty rate was 10.9% in 1985 and 13.5% in 2019 (Ministry of Health, Labour and Welfare, 2019) – which makes it likely today that one in seven children in Japan is living in poverty. The number of cases of reported child abuse has also risen. For a country that outwardly values children and families this is a significant concern.

In 2016, Japan's Child Welfare Law was significantly amended to clarify the principles for guaranteeing the welfare of children. Researchers working with children welcomed this change. Before these amendments, Article 1 of the Child Welfare Law stated:

> Every citizen shall endeavor to ensure that children are born healthy in mind and body and that they are nurtured' and every child shall be equally provided for and cared for.
>
> *Child Welfare Act (1948)*

However, after the amendments, the Article changed in its expression and now stated:

> Every child shall have the right, in the spirit of the UN Convention on the Rights of the Child, to be properly cared for, to have his or her life guaranteed, to be loved and protected, to have his or her physical and mental growth and development as well as his or her independence, and to have his or her welfare equally guaranteed.
>
> *Child Welfare Act, Article 1*

Before the changes to the Law, the subject was 'every citizen', implying that the focus of the law was the responsibility of adults and not necessarily the welfare of children. After the amendment, the subject was changed to 'every child' and it became clear for whom the law was intended.

UN Convention on the Rights of the Child

The UN Convention on the Rights of the Child (UNCRC) is probably familiar legislation in Western and European countries. However, children's rights are not commonly discussed in the care of sick children in Japan and there seems to be a lack of awareness of the UNCRC among medical professionals. It is important that HPSs spread the word that the UNCRC exists since it has such potential to positively impact children's lives.

The importance to see the child, not the diagnosis

When I teach student HPSs, I tell them not to think about one type or one category of children, but to reach out to all children. The reason why I teach students to think about every child, each in so many unique situations, is because I believe HPSs must not categorise children by condition like other medical professionals seem to do. It is not about how many tubes are coming out of the body, or what they look like, whether they can communicate verbally, or how many years they have left to live. We are the professionals who find and work with the child itself within the human body in front of us. We are professionals who will always try to connect with the child's spirit, which is sometimes hidden behind sickness or disability.

Our professional identity lies in how we play. As professionals we are expected to explain why we play with children and why children should play. However, the value of play has been trivialised in Japan, as in many other countries around the world. In 2010, the International Play Association identified the following ten barriers towards children playing in Tokyo.

- Lack of adult awareness of the importance of play
- Dangerous environment
- Parental anxiety
- Inadequate places and facilities to play
- Concerns about litigation
- Excessive pressure on children's academic performance
- Lack of awareness and facilities for children's play in schools
- Structured and programmed free time
- The high-tech and commercialisation of children's play
- The environment for children living in institutions

Takeda (2021)

While this list is from a playwork point of view, some points – specifically the lack of adult awareness of the importance of play, the structured and programmed free time and the environment for children living in institutions – are very common issues about which HPSs need awareness.

In *Homo Ludens*, Johan Huizinga (1971) expressed that "a culture that lacks the spirit of play is unworthy of its name, and a culture that has lost play is in danger of decadence" (p. 226). I believe the world of medicine contains its own culture – one dominated by a desire for children to live and – if they are sick – to be made well. If this is so, based on Huizinga's writing, the world of paediatrics needs to rethink its understanding of play. Play should be held in higher esteem because play itself is central to children's lives. Therefore, we need to think seriously about how to unite the worlds of medicine and children. We need to focus on the philosophy of hospital play and define it. My observation is that an increase in the number of adults who do not understand play leads to an increase in the number of children who cannot play. And my question in response is what kind of society will be formed by children who cannot play? I imagine it to be a very intolerant society in which children in need of medical care would be at risk. This is why HPSs must think about the welfare of all children and safeguard their emotional, psychological and moral well-being, as well as their physical health.

TSUBASA – A CHILD WHO CAME BACK TO HIS CHILDHOOD

Tsubasa experienced hypoxic encephalopathy as a result of an operation he underwent in the first year of primary school. This left him with paralysed limbs and he was unable to stand. He also needed regular suction, and spent most of the day in bed, connected to machines monitoring his heartbeat and vital signs.

Three years after his initial operation, I met Tsubasa. His mother showed me into the room, and I saw Tsubasa lying on a bed at the end of the room. Even from a distance, I could sense that he was a little nervous. There was a quietness, a sadness and a sense of resignation.

I walked straight over. I looked him in the eye, and I introduced myself. I said quietly, "Hello. I'm Chika and I'm here to play with Tsubasa". Tsubasa had a tracheotomy and was unable to speak. But he stared back at me. He looked at me intently and moved his lips very hard as if he was trying to answer me. I talked to Tsubasa a lot. I asked him what he liked to do for fun, just like any other child with a voice. I asked him about his schoolwork and about his family and his friends. Tsubasa didn't answer aloud, but he did move his eyes, flutter his eyelids and tried his best to move his mouth. I continued to chat with Tsubasa, responding to his silent answers. Tsubasa was very eloquent and the more we chatted, the more I could see (as I often told his parents) that Tsubasa's head was moving. His face became fearless. I could see that Tsubasa had a strong will. Tsubasa was talking so much that his father came to check on him. He saw a look on Tsubasa's face that said, "Don't interrupt me".

After about 20 minutes, Tsubasa started to doze off and my first visit was over (see Figures 24.1 and 24.2). I said to his parents, "I am so happy to have played with Tsubasa. To me, Tsubasa is like any fourth-grade boy".

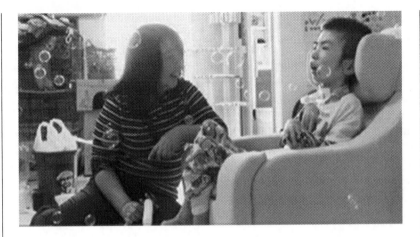

FIGURE 24.1 Tsubasa's bubbles.

I had enjoyed playing with Tsubasa and I couldn't wait to play with him again. My playful approach was very refreshing for the parents. It was the beginning of a journey for the parents and they both began to understand the value of bringing Hospital Play to Tsubasa. As a result, they gradually changed their approach to their son. They had a strong sense of remorse, because Tsubasa was once a healthy boy, running around. The sense of disappointment that I had felt in the whole room on my first visit was, in fact,

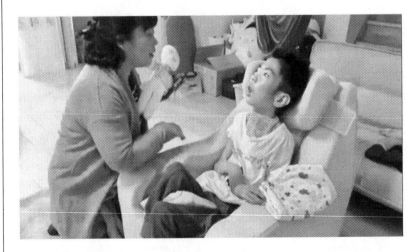

FIGURE 24.2 Tsubasa's doll.

the whole family's feelings about their situation. However, I observed that as Tsubasa began to play again, the following changes happened:

- Firstly, they saw their son as a child again, not as a sick child on a respirator. Many adults do not realise the important value of play, but through play Tsubasa's parents found a way to reconnect with their son.
- Secondly, Tsubasa was more able to express himself in a very rich way through play. His parents thought they would never be able to connect with Tsubasa, because he had no words. However, play is an important tool for communication.
- Third was a sense of hope. This is because play is fun in the first place. Through play, Tsubasa has experienced and enjoyed a great variety of games. For example, while reading the book *Going on a Bear Hunt*, Tsubasa stepped on the fallen leaves he had picked up with his feet. This was a bit scary for him. He hadn't stepped on anything with the soles of his feet for three years! However, when it was a game, he bravely tried. Tsubasa was determined to put his feet down and feel the leaves under his feet. The parents could see that change and that he was strong enough to live. The sight of Tsubasa playing gave them hope.
- Lastly, the change was joy. When Tsubasa was happy, his mother and father were happy too. It created a positive and cheerful atmosphere that swept away the shadow that had fallen over the family.

Conclusion

When the Hospital Play education course started, I was specialising in health systems research. I observed:

> When you go to a children's hospital … [and] you go into the room, it's dark and the only sound is the breathing apparatus. There will be several children lying there … When you look at them, you see their eyes moving. You ask the nurse "When do these children play?" She looks surprised and cannot answer. You need to have them playing. When that time comes you can say you have succeeded.
>
> *Matsudaira (2010, p. 4)*

Fifteen years have passed and so, we ask: Have the children in medical care in Japan been helped to play?

In 15 years, 214 HPSs have been trained and are now practising in hospitals around the country, making a difference for children in hospital in Japan. To go from no hospital play programmes at all to having HPSs working in almost every district of Japan is a significant achievement for a small profession, over a relatively short period of time. However, these practitioners work against the odds in a society that is failing to protect its children from living in poverty, as well as a medical system that struggles to value the basics of play even within children's normal development.

Over the next 15 years, further developments will be needed to strengthen the profession and to ensure that children – children like Tsubasa – continue to have opportunities to play, and by doing so to develop, and experience reconnection, communication, hope and joy during their hospital care. To achieve this goal, we certainly need to increase evidence of our work through academic research. It is also important to share the values of our HPS profession to other healthcare professionals to ensure the needs of children are firmly in the centre of their care. The devotion of Japanese HPSs – a small, growing and very dedicated group of professionals – has brought us to where we are now and will carry us forward into the future.

References

Huizinga, J. (1971) *Homo Ludens: A Study of the Play Element in Culture* (translated into Japanese from the original 1938 text by Kawade, Shobou). Tokyo: Sinshya.

Matsudaira, C. (2010) *Introduction to Hospital Play*. Tokyo: Kenpakusha.

Ministry of Health, Labour and Welfare (2019) *Overview of the 2019 National Survey of Living Standards. Status of Poverty Rates' Table 11 and Figure 13: Annual Trends in Poverty Rates*. p. 14. [Online] Available from: <https://www.mhlw.go.jp/toukei/saikin/hw/k-tyosa/k-tyosa19/dl/03.pdf> [Accessed 4 August 2022].

Takeda, N. (2021) *Yarisugi Kyouiku*. Tokyo: Popuro Shobou.

25

LET'S START WITH PLAY

Why play in the Emergency Department can be our best tool for interventions

Cala Hefferan – Certified Child Life Specialist

Laura Sufka – Certified Child Life Specialist

For many children, a visit to the Emergency Department can be extremely frightening and overwhelming. The pediatric patient often enters the Emergency Department experiencing stress, trauma, fear, and misconceptions. During heightened stress, child life specialists assess pediatric patients' natural coping techniques. Child life specialists partner with patients and their families to appraise the situation and identify natural coping strategies. Engaging in play with pediatric patients in the Emergency Department can normalise the environment as the pediatric patient processes and appraises potential stressors (Yogman et al., 2018). Child life specialists witness the power of play not as a distraction but rather as a buffer that neutralises potential stress and trauma, affording pediatric patients a more recognisable environment.

Established in play, natural coping techniques build trust and rapport to create a safe environment. Play is powerful and radiates from within a child, bridging communication and supporting learning. Play is crucial to a child's social, emotional, and cognitive development and is even more critical during times of adversity or stress (Yogman et al., 2018). Pediatric patients gravitate towards play, allowing for successful adaptation within an environment where they have little control, thus strengthening resilience.

The following reflection demonstrates how play mediates pediatric medical stress for patients in the Emergency Department (names have been changed to protect the confidentiality of our patients and families).

On this particular day, I was working in the Pediatric Emergency Department. I closely monitored the coming and going of nurses and doctors, paying close attention to how patients and families were coping when I noticed a little girl carried by a man into our Emergency Department. The man quietly spoke to

DOI: 10.4324/9781003255444-30

the little girl in Spanish as the staff quickly led him into their assigned room. I swiftly and intentionally walked towards the room, ears, and eyes alert, assessing her efforts to cope and the man's body disposition while navigating the emergency department environment. I quickly assessed the patient's developmental level, stress potential, and family presence and comfort in navigating the Emergency Department experience (Burns-Nader & Hernandez-Reif, 2016). As I listened patiently and intently, I assessed the impact of this experience on this pediatric patient while considering how I could collaborate with my colleagues to best support coping so as to minimize stress and trauma.

As I walked up to the room, checking my bag for age-appropriate items, I intently listened and quickly gathered the last bits of information. I could hear the urgency in the nurse's voice as she attempted to take the patient's vitals. The little girl sounded inconsolable, and as I turned into the room, I could see the man's bewildered eyes as his gaze caught my attention, pulling me closer. It was clear that this duo and the Emergency Department staff would benefit from child life support in navigating this patient's Emergency Department experience.

From my brief observations, I assessed that the patient was about four years of age, inconsolable, preferred to be close to the man carrying her, and likely was experiencing an allergic reaction. The man (perhaps her father) spoke Spanish and demonstrated some understanding and ability to communicate in English. Considering my assessment, I entered the room. I introduced myself and my role while assessing the man's understanding of English and offering to call a phone interpreter while carefully respecting the little girl's preference for me to stay away from her. The man introduced himself as Santiago, the girl's father, and thanked me for offering an interpreter but that he did not need one at this time. Then, Santiago began sharing the situation leading to his daughter coming to the Emergency Department. Santiago shared that Abigail, his daughter, was ill after eating peanut butter.

With the knowledge from my initial assessment of observation and conversation with Abigail's father, I adjusted the head of the bed to support a seated position. I helped Santiago comfortably sit on the bed with Abigail in his arms. Abigail made it very clear she preferred to be chest to chest with her father. The nurse nodded in approval that this position would work just fine, and I communicated to Santiago that we could care for Abigail while they remained chest to chest. Once Santiago and Abigail were seated, I quickly scanned the room, looking for a bag with comfort items for Abigail from home. Noticing a large bag, I inquired if Abigail's favorite toys or comfort items were in the bag. Santiago shared that Abigail's favorite book was in the bag, but her favorite stuffed animal was in the car because she vomited on it during the car ride. I offered to read the book to Abigail as she rested in her father's arms. Abigail snuggled in her father's arms and, crying, nodded her head. I started reading the book to Abigail, and she intently listened. Her cries turned to whimpers with time, and her body slowly relaxed into her father's arms.

Knowing that vitals needed to occur and that the doctor urgently needed to examine Abigail, I started to relate parts of the objects in the book to the room to support the normalization of the room and people. I shared that Nancy, Abigail's nurse, would use her stethoscope, a special microphone that nurses and doctors use to listen to our breathing and heartbeat, to listen to Abigail's heart and lungs today.

As I continued to describe the equipment and use developmentally appropriate words, I offered Abigail choices and chances to exert autonomy. Abigail chose to hold the stethoscope so the doctor could listen to her father's heart and then again as the doctor listened to her heart. Medical play afforded Abigail a sense of control, allowing her a safe space to express her feelings and increase her understanding (Burns-Nader & Hernandez-Reif, 2016; Jones, 2018). I continued to support Abigail's coping by playfully engaging in one particular page of the book, where the main character was dressed as a doctor. Abigail's favorite book became the backdrop from which the medical team could assess and medically treat her with the swiftness and urgency needed. At the same time, I continued to focus on lessening the stressfulness of the situation for Abigail and her father.

The play-based interventions, including normative and medical play decreased Abigail's anxiety, allowed a safe space for expressing feelings, and provided opportunities for Abigail to exert control. As research and experience demonstrate, play-based interventions can buffer the potential trauma of the Emergency Department visit by normalizing the environment and allowing the pediatric patient to feel more comfortable, appraise the situation as one they can have some control over, and regulate the body's stress response (Burns-Nader & Hernandez-Reif, 2016; Yogman et al., 2018).

Partnering with families is essential to facilitating play-based interventions that support pediatric patients (American Academy of Pediatrics, 2021). When supporting Abigail's coping in the Emergency Department, I partnered with Santiago acknowledging that Santiago truly knew Abigail best. I have often seen when a caregiver's expertise and ability to support pediatric patient coping has gone unacknowledged or unsupported, resulting in the caregiver feeling helpless and the child feeling frightened and alone. It is the pivotal work of the child life specialist to acknowledge the dynamic relationship between caregiver and child and empower the caregiver's ability to comfort and support their child during their Emergency Department experience (American Academy of Pediatrics, 2021). Assessing the natural play interactions that sustain the caregiver and child connection and then demonstrating and empowering caregivers and patients to utilize these play-based interactions to support coping is at the core of play-based interventions. When working with Abigail and Santiago, I assessed that reading Abigail's favorite book was a play interaction that supported the patient and caregiver connection and Abigail's coping ability.

Once Santiago appeared calm and had time to adjust to this new experience, we transitioned to Santiago reading the book to Abigail. My actions affirmed that the play interaction of reading together at home was welcome here in the emergency department to support Abigail's coping. Next, my role transitioned to ensuring Santiago had what he needed to support Abigail confidently. I provided Santiago with a stuffed animal to give to Abigail and a fresh change of clothes. As Santiago and Abigail continued to navigate how to cope with this new environment, I observed Santiago's phone ringing. I inquired, and Santiago shared that his wife had been calling as she was worried about Abigail but that he (Santiago) could not hold the phone and Abigail and the book. I offered to hold the phone so that Abigail could video chat with her mother to continue to support the caregiver and pediatric patient connection. As a result, Abigail's mom sang a song to Abigail while she took her medicine ordered by the doctor, just as they did at home when taking medication. I am happy to report that when Abigail left the Emergency Department later that night, she walked with confidence holding her father's hand and her new stuffed animal smiling and waving "goodbye" to staff.

Cala Hefferan – Fall (2021)

As we continue to imagine utilising play in the Emergency Department, let's take a minute to ponder a question. Can you imagine walking into a new room, not knowing anyone, and not even entirely sure why you are there? How do you alert your body and mind that it is ok? You look for things, people, and items that alert you to feel safe. Before any conversations or procedures can happen, we must gain the child's trust. Otherwise, we are attempting to give the child information they may not process or listen to because their more significant concern is if they can trust the person giving them this information. We suggest merely beginning the encounter with play, communicating that we are present to meet the patient where they are at; that we are willing to step into their shoes; that we are interested in better understanding their fears, worries, and misconceptions. Truly, taking this brief moment to meet a child with a playful interaction communicates a deep level of caring and thus builds trust. When children identify a person as safe, they may share their concerns, fears, and questions (Gordon & Paisley, 2018). As a child life specialist, play allows us to enter this situation. It enables us to walk into a room where a child has never met us and alert them that we are on their team. We must challenge ourselves to see the child first and the illness or injury second as child life specialists.

Sometimes play is not a toy or item but rather a playful interaction between caregiver and child. Even if a child can't engage in play at first, watching an adult play may promote play in the future. As child life specialists, we can equip caregivers to reimagine how playful interactions can translate and support their child during an Emergency Department visit. Depending on the child's age, the child may be unsure if the adult is a helper or someone who may bring harm to them. Similarly, many caregivers can remember negative experiences they had as a child. When caregivers enter the Emergency Department, their anxiety may increase, and their ability to provide comfort to their child may become difficult. Past emergency room visits can have trauma reminders not only for our minds but also for our bodies (Woodburn et al., 2020). Play gives the child the ability to alleviate the stress experienced in this unfamiliar environment, calm their body, gain the trust of the medical team, and then listen to the new information related to the procedure or treatment plan. Play, specifically playful interactions, may also calm the caregiver. A moment of play allows the caregiver to reappraise the situation and tap into their innate abilities. Caregivers generally know how to calm and comfort their children and can be pivotal to ensuring the best emergency room experience for their child (Kuttner, 1996).

The following reflection demonstrates how play mediates pediatric medical stress for patients in the Emergency Department.

> I can see her entering through the double doors – the nurse leading the way. Mom gently holds her daughter's arm as she cries out in pain. She is about two years old. I have enough time to grab a small magic wand and bubbles. The doctor and I enter the room. The doctor places herself across the room but is still eye to eye with the mom. No one is speaking except for the loud cries of the child. Is she in pain, scared of her new environment, or both? I slowly move farther away from the child but still engage the child with my eyes. I am in her space, so I wait to be invited closer. Children already come to us with coping abilities or tools; build off those. In this situation, this child's greatest coping tool is to stay as close to her mom as possible. She cries and pulls at her mom to hold her closer as the doctor examines her arm with only her eyes. Then she spots them, the bubbles. Play has begun. By starting with play, we are truly meeting the needs of a child. Play equalizes the room. If we center the child and keep our agenda child-driven instead of adult-driven, we would utilize play as our first tool of engagement.
>
> Bubbles slowly fall from the ceiling to the floor. Intentionally I continue to shower the ceiling with bubbles. The bubbles fall slowly and gently, hopefully becoming synced with the child's breathing and the possibility of the child grabbing for them. Grabbing would allow our assessment of the arm to continue. But she's not ready yet; still unsure of this new environment and the people within her space. In my experience, rushing any child will only decrease their ability to cope and master their healthcare experience, and overall the procedure will take longer. Within minutes her breathing slowed, and her cries lessened. I continue to blow and now catch the bubbles with my bubble wand. I offer the bubble. Hoping she will reach with her hand to pop it. It would be her way of telling me, "It is ok to enter my space now". She pops it with the arm that she isn't protecting. While the child and I continue to pop bubbles, the doctor

can engage the mom in conversation. When did this happen? How did it happen? Does it appear that she hurt anything else besides her arm? It is clear that mom's breathing has also slowed down, and she can engage with the doctor. As I build rapport and trust with the child, she begins to laugh and shows signs of trusting us. She isn't moving her one arm, but she is now sitting independently on the bed with mom close to her side and fully engaging in play with me.

The next step is to take an X-ray of the arm. Mom verbalizes concern that the patient won't be able to sit still for the X-ray and will probably have increased anxiety due to separation. I gathered a stuffed animal, medical play supplies, and pictures of the X-ray machine. Intentionally exploring and playing with medical equipment (e.g., masks, gloves, syringes, and stethoscopes) is an essential component of children's coping in health care settings. Combining recognizable play methods (e.g., non-scripted and intrinsically motivated play) and unfamiliar medical equipment allows children the opportunity to integrate their thoughts and feelings regarding the situation (Bolig, 2018; Jones, 2018).

When the medical play session begins, the child plays through her experience exploring the stethoscope and other items. The patient uses the stuffed animal as her patient. While I prepare the mom for the X-ray with verbal explanations, pictures, and developmentally appropriate coping at this age, I utilize the stuffed animal to model sitting on the mom's lap for the X-ray. The stuffed animal sits on mom's lap. I use a magic wand and light spinner to model how the patient could engage in play and distraction while having an X-ray – encouraging the stuffed animal to "stay still like a statue" and "wiggle its toes" if it feels like it needs to move its body. Research has demonstrated that children are less fearful and distressed when positioned for medical procedures in a sitting position rather than supine (Lacey, Finkelstein, & Thygeson, 2008).

Now it is time for the patient to practice sitting on mom's lap. With the help of her mom (protecting the arm), the patient can sit in her mom's lap while holding the stuffed animal. I engage the child in the light spinner and sing the 'Wheels on the Bus' song, modelling to the mom ways to support her child during an X-ray. I encourage the mom to guide the child through the X-ray using words and songs familiar to the child. Due to the ever-changing needs of the emergency department throughout each shift, if a patient and caregiver's assessment shows signs of coping and mastery before a radiology procedure, I will not accompany them to the room where the procedure will be taking place.

The child and mom returned from the X-ray, reporting that the light-up spinner worked great to distract the child and engage her enough to sit still for the arm X-ray. I find this debriefing just as critical as the preparation for any procedure. This time allows me to validate a caregiver and help them recognize their extraordinary ability to support their child in this fast-paced and sometimes overwhelming environment. They truly know their child the very best and can utilize those intuitive skills to help their child. For a child, this time also allows for continued medical play and mastery over their experience while waiting for the radiology results.

After the doctor examined the X-ray, it was determined that the child had a minor fracture. In our emergency department, we use a splint to stabilize the fracture and then have the family follow up with a pediatric orthopedic doctor after a few days, and the swelling has lessened. Because I was able to introduce medical play earlier in the visit, I just gathered a few additional items for her to explore. I gently slide a chair next to the bed where she is already playing with the medical play supplies and invites me into her space, holding up the stethoscope to try on. I began modelling but allowed her to control the play on the stuffed animal and verbally explain to mom the next steps. Allowing the child to pick which arm to measure and wrap the soft bandage around. The child quickly engages and asks her mom to help wrap the bandage around the arm.

As child life specialists, we work to empower and equip caregivers with tools and suggestions for future healthcare experiences when a child life specialist may not be present. By engaging caregivers in the medical play process, child life specialists have the opportunity to educate and empower caregivers to understand more of the internal landscape of their child's coping and engage with them in a way that supports ongoing emotional expression and mastery of their emergency room experiences (Rubin, 2018). As we finish our medical play session, a nursing assistant enters the room to set up the splint materials. At this time, I introduce the next therapeutic play opportunity. While mom sits on the bed with her child in between her lap in an upright position, I place myself next to the child but on the opposite side of the fractured arm. As the bed moves up, I raise a magic wand towards the ceiling and engage the child in a musical tune to distract and engage the child in play, as transitions can be difficult at this age. The child reaches for the wand and grabs it with her non-fractured arm. The nursing assistant is ready to begin splinting and engage in the gentle dance of placing a splint on the child's arm while I engage the child in placing a splint on her stuffed animal. With the help and support of mom and me, the child measures the stuffed animal's arm, places a splint, and then decorates the splint with stickers, all while having a splint placed on her fractured arm. Following the splint placement, she picked up her stuffed animal and showed it to everyone in the room, and said, "like me".

Laura Sufka – December (2019)

We must challenge ourselves and those we work with to reframe our thinking from "this child is coming to the emergency department today and only today" to "this child is here today and will likely have future visits to the emergency department or healthcare facilities". Acknowledging the bigger picture for the child propels us to align our actions with building resiliency because of awareness of the negative impacts of pediatric medical trauma. Each child and family entering these spaces comes with a level of trauma that they have already experienced in their life. However, providing appropriate choices and expression of feelings affords children a sense of mastery and control over their healthcare experience. Child life specialists and other healthcare providers have the opportunity to minimise the potentially traumatic aspects of medical care and identify children and families with pediatric medical traumatic stress. Pediatric medical traumatic stress encompasses a set of psychological and physiological responses to potentially traumatic events such as pain, injury, serious illness, medical procedures, and invasive or frightening treatment experiences (National Child Traumatic Stress Network, 2003).

Providing play from the very beginning and throughout an emergency room visit can address the potential for additional medical traumatic stress. Transitioning play from the Emergency Department to the child's home can provide additional benefits to a child's long-term coping. When children are in the safety of their home, they start to make sense of their entire experience. They may gather their toys or stuffed animals and engage in medical play freely. Playing a vital role in this is the caregiver who just went through this emergency room visit with the child. However exhausted or relieved you and your child may feel, sharing your experiences with each other in the aftermath of an emergency may be as important as, or even more important than, what went on during the experience itself, especially if the experience was more negative than what you would have liked (Kuttner, 1996). One way child life specialists encourage continued processing of their medical experiences is to provide medical play kits for children to take home. Medical play and materials specific to the child's treatment give children access to play with medical themes and medical equipment offered in a non-threatening manner (Woodburn et al., 2020). Children can play out feelings and thoughts about their recent emergency room visit by continuing processing at home. Research indicates that children who play with items related to their stressors experience reduced anxiety and greater coping ability (Woodburn et al., 2020). In addition, caregivers are also given a front-row seat into their child's experiences and become more aware of their child's feelings and possible misconceptions of their emergency room visit. As child life specialists, we know every emergency room experience is different. Therefore, we can support coping, resilience, competence, and growth and provide anticipatory guidance to prevent long-lasting traumatic stress reactions (Stenman et al., 2019).

In acknowledging and accepting the power of play, child life specialists validate and advocate for play opportunities. Play interventions (including medical play, creative arts, and age-appropriate distraction) support communication, promote resiliency, and allow children to feel empowered and gain ownership over their medical experiences within the pediatric Emergency Department. In addition, as children master their world, play aids in the development of new competencies that lead to enhanced confidence and the resiliency they will need to face future challenges (American Academy of Pediatrics, 2007).

Therefore, we posit it is crucial that as child life specialists and advocates for play, we continue to ask ourselves, "How can I reimagine and incorporate the importance of play into the emergent needs of pediatric patients in the emergency department?"

References

American Academy of Pediatrics (2007) The importance of play in promoting healthy child development and maintaining strong parent-child bonds, *Pediatrics*, 119 (1), pp. 182–191

American Academy of Pediatrics (2021) Policy statement: Child life services, *Pediatrics*, 147 (1)

Bolig, R. (2018) Play in Children's Health-Care Settings. In: Rollins, J., Bolig, R. & Mahan, C. (Eds.) *Meeting Children's Psychosocial Needs across the Health-care Continuum* (pp. 77–117). Austin, TX: Pro-Ed, Inc.

Burns-Nader, S. & Hernandez-Reif, M. (2016) Facilitating play for hospitalized children through child life services, *Children's Health Care*, 45 (1), pp. 1–21

Gordon, J. & Paisley, S. (2018) Trauma-Focused Medical Play. In: Rubin, L.C. (Ed.) *Handbook of Medical Play Therapy and Child Life: Interventions in Clinical and Medical Settings.* New York, NY: Routledge

Jones, M. (2018) The necessity of play in healthcare settings, *Pediatric Nursing*, 44 (6) pp. 303–305

Kuttner, L. (1996) *A Child in Pain: How to Help, What to Do.* Carmarthen: Crown House Publishing

Lacey, C., Finkelstein, M., & Thygeson, M. (2008) The impact of positioning on fear during immunizations: Supine versus sitting up, *Journal of Pediatric Nursing*, 23 (3), pp. 195–200

National Child Traumatic Stress Network (2003) What Is Child Traumatic Stress? *Claiming Children*. [Online] Available from: <https://www.nctsn.org/sites/default/files/resources//what_is_child_traumatic_stress.pdf> [Accessed 4 May 2022]

Rubin, L. (ed.) (2018) *Handbook of Medical Play Therapy and Child Life: Interventions in Clinical and Medical Settings.* New York, NY: Routledge

Stenman, K., Christofferson, J., Alderfer, M., Pierce, J., Kelly, C., Schifano, E., Klaff, S., Sciolla, J., Deatrick, J., & Kazak, A. (2019) Integrating play in trauma-informed care: Multidisciplinary pediatric healthcare provider perspectives, *Psychological Services*, 16 (1), pp. 7–15

Woodburn, A., Munn, E., Jones, M., Hoskins, K., Gill, M., Fraser, C., Dunbar, J., Duplechain, A., Boles, J., & Bennett, K. (2020) The Value of Certified Child Life Specialists: Direct and Downstream Optimization of Pediatric Patient and Family Outcomes. *Association of Child Life Professionals*. [Online] Available from: < https://www.childlife.org/docs/default-source/the-child-life-profession/value-of-cclss-full-report.pdf> [Accessed 4 May 2022]

Yogman, M., Garner A., Hutchinson, J., Hirsh-Pasek, K., & Golinkoff R. (2018) The power of play: A pediatric role in enhancing development in young children, *Pediatrics*, 142 (3), pp. 1–16

PART V

Playing in other ways and other settings

26

PLAY IN A CHILDREN'S HOSPICE ...
WHAT IS THE POINT?

*Lynda Elliott – Play Team Co-ordinator
and Outreach Specialist*

The hospice is a 12-bed, nurse-led unit, offering planned short breaks, palliative and symptom control admissions and end of life care, for babies, children and young people, who have life-limiting/threatening conditions. This broad umbrella guarantees there is a wide range of ages, interests, abilities and personalities resident at any one time. In addition, to this we also offer some outreach support for some families within the community.

Play is an integral part of that support, but why? After all the child is dying, so what is the point ...?

It is simply not enough to state, "because, as we know, play is important".

Article 31 of the United Convention on the Rights of the Child states that "every child has the right to rest, relax, play and take part in cultural and creative activities" (UNICEF 1991). This is still relevant if a child has a medical condition, complex sensory impairments, time-consuming care requirements or is dying.

Play in a children's hospice inevitably includes activities that help to create memories, some occur quite naturally, others take more planning and time, but all will be unique to individual families.

Over the years I have been able to facilitate numerous different sessions, including taking lots of photographs, family film evenings, a New Year party, birthday celebrations, Christmas in July, a trip to feed the ducks, creating a beach in our multi-sensory room (complete with fishy smells), assisting with writing letters and making gifts for family members, taking prints for jewellery or tattoos, hand and foot casts and my personal favourite of encouraging family members to create a collage of their hand/finger/foot prints (Figure 26.1).

DOI: 10.4324/9781003255444-32

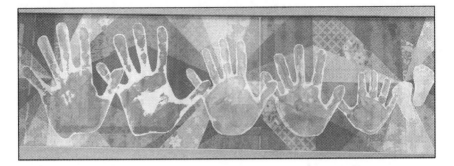

FIGURE 26.1 Handprints.

MINI CASE STUDY 1

B was 16 years old when I met him; he had a rare and degenerative condition, which was affecting him both physically and cognitively. There was a family history of this condition and B was fully aware of his future prognosis.

B had a rapid deterioration, meaning he was unable to attend school and spent the majority of his time within the family home. That was when I received the referral for Play/Activities input and emotional support.

The initial sessions focused on activities he might enjoy to ensure that he had a positive focus in his day, which had nothing to do with his condition or any limitations he was experiencing. Early sessions were often art and craft based as this was what B liked to do most. I needed to adapt some of the equipment he used to make sure he was able to be as independent as possible. I took a variety of activities to do so that B had a choice. I also found some permanent marker pens that could be erased (if wiped quickly enough) so that if B was to experience his frequent, involuntary "jerky" movements whilst crafting, the marks made could be removed. During these sessions B made gifts for many members of his family.

I began taking a range of activities with me, as B's condition was quite unpredictable – sometimes I read to him and played different types of music if he was having a number of seizures and feeling quite unwell. Art and craft remained a firm favourite and this would often be when B would chat about all sorts of things. We would explore different emotions and feelings we experience generally, through games, and gradually this became the time he would talk about family members that had died, and ultimately his own life.

His condition continued to deteriorate and he became more confused and sleepier during our sessions, so we moved to more sensory activities including hand massage, I always offered a choice of creams and asked B to choose which he preferred. Towards the end of one of our sessions where B had been mostly passive, I asked if he would like to select a cream, after smelling the two I offered, he smiled, looked directly at me and said "I remember who you are now". We always started future sessions with the creams, by way of introducing myself.

Initially my role was to facilitate activities that B enjoyed, this meant looking at his interests and seeing what adaptations might be possible for him to maintain his skills for as long as possible. Finding the simple resource of pens that wiped away, if corrected immediately, had a fantastic positive benefit on B's self-esteem – any "mistakes" that were made could be erased. Prior to this he would have focused on these marks, highlighting how he was deteriorating.

B chose to gift many of his art creations to family members, creating a legacy as he was fully aware of his prognosis. Foster et al. (2012) talk about (memory) legacy-making enhancing the life of and decreasing suffering for dying children and their families and go on to suggest that this can confirm the child is loved and will be remembered. Many children need and want to know that they will not be forgotten.

Using the activities that B enjoyed during the initial sessions enabled us to move naturally onto the subject of his feelings and emotions around his condition and previous family bereavements. It was important that this space remained within B's control but with opportunities to think about and discuss challenging issues. "Since the children interpret death as an inappropriate topic of conversation with adults" (Bluebond-Langner 1978, pg 10) and "Children may also try to protect the adults around them from further pain ... they may suppress their need to cry and act out their distress" (Smith 1999 pg 16). This was particularly true for B.

I was aware that B's condition was deteriorating and that some of his presentation resembled dementia, but at the end of the session after smelling the hand creams, he was able to remember who I was. That really highlighted the power of our senses in recalling memories and absolutely influenced my practice moving forward.

MINI CASE STUDY 2

I met D and his parents when they arrived at the hospice, as it was believed that D's life would be significantly shortened following a very traumatic birth and subsequent hospitalisation in a Neonatal Intensive Care Unit. Although he continued to be a very poorly baby, with very complex and medically challenging needs, after three weeks at Rainbows his parents were supported to care for him at home.

D was referred to me for some Outreach Play sessions to support Mum with "stimulation, activity ideas and confidence building".

Following an assessment visit, I suggested I could visit regularly, focusing on sensory experiences based around a theme or story. It was challenging to assess D's enjoyment level, however his breathing changed and his facial expressions allowed me to judge if he **wasn't** happy, so became my benchmark. Mum became very involved during our sessions and I would usually leave the story book and resources I had used, as she was keen to repeat the sessions herself – they developed a routine whereby D would have a bedtime story every evening. Mum also encouraged members of their extended family to use the stories and materials as a way of engaging with D as they were also struggling to interact in a meaningful way with him.

During our Christmas session I used a painted footprint of D's to make a Christmas card for Mummy and Daddy and although this proved to be very emotional for Mum to receive, she asked if I could leave the paints for her to use ... the following day she sent me a photograph of a selection of cards she and Aunty had helped D to make, for lots of family members.

After a while D's parents' work commitments changed and Dad became D's full-time carer as Mum returned to work. My visits continued and Dad was as enthusiastic to join in with the sensory play sessions.

On one very special visit I was able to support them in making a family hand-cast – all three of them held hands and a mould was created, then filled with plaster to capture their imprints.

Shortly after that visit D and his parents came to stay at the hospice for a planned visit; he seemed "a little under the weather" according to Mum. He had a sensory bath and went out into our garden for a while, where he died very peacefully. The family stayed at the hospice with D until his funeral where the wider team supported his parents and ensured D's body was suitably cared for. D's parents asked if it would be possible to capture casts of his feet, I was able to offer this and with both Mum and Dad present we were able to create the moulds and ultimately the casts.

At D's funeral, family members talked about the time they had spent with D, many voicing how precious their Christmas cards that he had made were, but possibly more importantly, his cousins talked about how they had loved to read D his stories, using the "funny items" that I had put together to go with the story.

Looking back on my interactions with D and his family it is really easy for me to think "this is just what I do", but on reflection there are clearly many elements to this. Firstly, it is about communication and forming a positive professional relationship, both with the baby and his parents. Spending time to establish any changes in facial expressions and breathing patterns for those children who have very complex needs is often the best way of assessing how they are feeling.

It is invaluable getting the family involved with activities; play needs to be an integral part of any child's experiences, not just when the Health Play Specialist is delivering a session. For this reason, I am very keen to supply and use every day, easy to source, reasonably priced items, showing how these can be used creatively and simply. This builds confidence for families to make play a 'normal' part of their child's routine. Hearing D's cousins talk at his funeral, reinforced, how important this type of interaction is amongst all children; they were able to join in and share D's play in a way that he was not able to participate in theirs.

Blower (2010 pg 174) touches on this, specifically referring to siblings. However, I feel this can be extended to all close children relatives:

> This means that they are often not spending quality time together ... doing activities that other families take for granted ... and do not have the type of relationship that their peers may have with theirs.

My sessions with children who have very complex needs often involve some form of art and craft. This is as a result of a parent telling me that a picture I "helped" a child to make out of lots of different textured materials we had spent the session exploring, was the first picture he had ever done, and he could now be like his brothers who had lots of artwork displayed on the kitchen cupboards.

Hand and footprints are unique and can be transformed into almost anything (Figure 26.2).

As mentioned previously, Foster et al. (2012) talk about (memory) legacy-making. They go on to suggest it is thought to benefit bereaved families and provides a tangible memento of their deceased child.

Spending time with a child after death can be incredibly important for parents in the process of their grief. Being able to support his parents by creating the casts of D's feet provided time and purpose for their interactions at a time filled with sadness and loss, as well as producing something tangible for them to continue to hold (Figure 26.3).

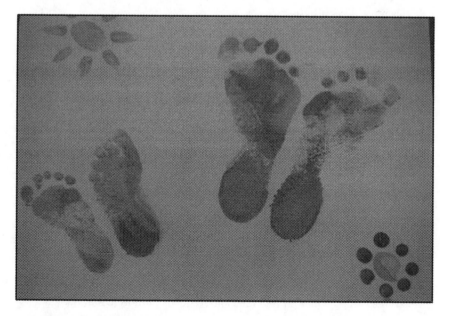

FIGURE 26.2 Footprints.

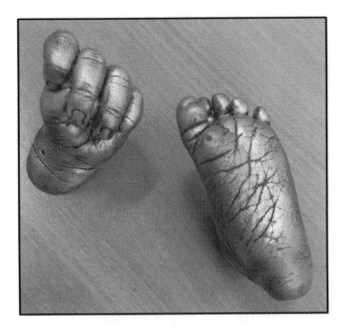

FIGURE 26.3 Hand and foot casts.

Van Aerde (2001) states that:

> Caregivers who provide this level of care will fulfil the unique needs of grieving parents by assisting them to have positive memories of their baby, and by giving them a feeling of being cared for in the midst of their pain and grief.

And Leon (1992) says:

> Bereaved parents never forget the understanding, respect, and genuine warmth they received from caregivers, which can become as lasting and important as any other memories of their lost pregnancy or their baby's brief life.

This is echoed, anecdotally, by many parents I have worked alongside.

MINI CASE STUDY 3

L is seven years old and has autism and a medical condition which means she is life limited and has prolonged and frequent seizures, behavioural and developmental delay, limited speech, a very short attention span, and whilst being fully ambulant, she has little/no awareness of her personal safety. This combination often results in L hearing "NO" and being redirected to something else.

L had been staying at the hospice for 2 days already as part of a planned short break and I was keen to provide an activity that was in a safe environment, stimulating and where she could have more freedom to explore. I decided to hold a painting session in a bathroom (L wore an adult size painting shirt, rather than her own clothes).

Initially L painted on the paper I had provided on the floor, but then this spilled over onto the floor. L was quiet, but appeared engaged. Gradually she appeared to become aware of the mirror ahead of her and she stood and moved closer and looked at her reflection. I asked L who could she see and she smiled. L then put the paintbrush onto the mirror and giggled, she turned to look at me and I smiled. I asked L if she wanted more paint and L replied "pink" (I was totally unaware that she could say this word – or indeed differentiate between colours).

I painted my hand and put a print on the wall. I asked L if she wanted to do the same, and she gave me her hand. I asked what colour she wanted me to used – she replied "purple". I picked up the yellow and asked if this was the colour she wanted – she frowned and repeated the word "purple", so I picked up the correct paint and helped L to cover her hand. L rubbed the paint in with her other hand and said "squishy" before putting her prints onto the wall next to mine. L continued to paint, reaching for different paints and saying the colours and used words like "more" and "gone" (when a bottle was empty). She poured some paint onto the mirror and watched it dribble down and repeated this a number of times, often passing me a bottle of paint and indicating for me to pour some on too. L continued to be chatty throughout and interacted positively, especially when other members of staff passed the bathroom and commented on her "masterpiece", she smiled and said "Look". I told L that when she had finished she could go for a bath (a favourite activity of L's).

I had anticipated that this activity would last only a short time – L continued with this activity for 55 minutes! She used far more language than I had been aware of and showed understanding of different concepts, e.g. gone, more, squishy and colour recognition.

L has been coming to the Hospice for planned short breaks for a while and the staff know her well. However, it can prove challenging for them to create opportunities for meaningful play due to the safety concerns, her concentration span, and her love of an iPad.

It was important to me that she should have as much freedom as possible during our session, as she regularly hears "No" and is redirected to a safer space throughout the day. The bathroom seemed to be the area that would be safe, offer her space and was the easiest to clean following our painting session.

The language and communication displayed during this session was far more complex than I had previously experienced from L, proving that when we join children in THEIR world, rather than expecting them to come into ours, it allows us to understand them far better. Bennie (2020) talks about developing joint attention:

> Joint attention means both the adult and the child are fixed on the same thing at the same time, experiencing the same reaction and awareness that both people are involved. This process takes time to develop in ASD. Beginning with creating a sense of shared space – sharing attention, emotion and understanding...Young autistic children tend to avoid sharing space, finding it uncomfortable...Try to start with sharing space, even if just for a few seconds, to show that it can be fun.

L concentrated on this activity for much longer than I had imagined and offering a bath at the end of the painting session meant there was still something positive to look forward to once the session finished and she was back with the care staff (Figure 26.4).

Traditionally, Health Play Specialists focus on three main areas: preparation, distraction and normalised play. In the Hospice, these are still integral to my

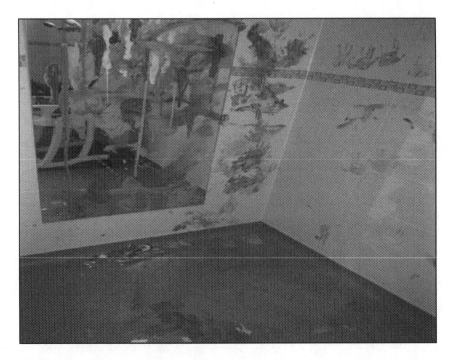

FIGURE 26.4 Painting session.

role. It is just that what is being prepared for, distracted from and normalised, includes death and dying.

Play provides:

- A language to communicate with, that is much more than verbal
- Control of a situation or time, when there seems to be very little that the child has in their control
- Opportunities to understand what is happening in their world and influence the outcomes
- Time to explore their thoughts, feelings and fears
- The chance to contribute and create their own legacies
- A space to "be" in the moment

So, what IS the point?

The point is, that the children and young people I work alongside still have their lives to live, communication to share, a legacy to build and the right to do so.

References

Bennie, M. (2020) The Importance of Play for Autistic Children. *Autism Awareness Centre Inc.* [Online blog]. Available from: < https://autismawarenesscentre.com/the-importance-of-play-for-children-with-asd/> [Accessed 12 March 2022]

Blower, S. (2010) Hearing the Voices of Siblings. In: Pfund, R. & Fowler-Kelly, S. *Perspectives on Palliative Care for Children and Young People.* Oxford: Radcliffe Publishing

Bluebond-Langner, M. (1978) *The Private Worlds of Dying Children.* Princeton, NJ: Princeton University Press

Foster, T., Dietrich, M., Friedman, D., Gordon, J. & Gilmer, M. (2012) National Survey of Children's Hospitals on Legacy-Making Activities. *Journal of Palliative Medicine*, Vol. 15. 5, pp. 573–578

Leon, I. (1992) Perinatal Loss: A Critique of Current Hospital Practices. *Clinical Pediatrics*, Vol. 31. 6, pp. 366–374

Smith, S. (1999) *The Forgotten Mourners.* London: Jessica Kingsley

UNICEF (1991) *United Nations Convention on the Rights of the Child.* Svenska: UNICEF Kommitten

Van Aerde, J. (2001) Guidelines for Health Care Professionals Supporting Families Experiencing a Perinatal Loss. *Paediatrics & Child Health*, Vol. 6. 7, pp. 469–477

27

THE THERAPEUTIC POWER OF PLAY FOR CHRONICALLY ABUSED CHILDREN

Fraser Brown – Emeritus Professor of Playwork and Childhood Development

Context

In the early 1990s, following the overthrow of the Romanian President, Nicolae Ceauşescu, the Western media began to gain access to the former communist state of Romania. They discovered a country whose institutions were substantially failing, partly because of the collapse of its financial systems, but largely because of the legacy of the Ceauşescu era (Deletant, 1995). In one of the poorest countries in Europe, Ceauşescu's people had been subjected to a raft of bizarre dictums. For example, he thought that building the country's industrial base would require an increase in the population. Therefore, contraception was banned for families with fewer than five children, and women were often medically 'examined' by a special branch of the police to make sure they were not having abortions (Gloviczki, 2004). As a result of these and other factors, more than a hundred thousand children were living in orphanages (Nelson et al., 2014). Many were HIV+, which meant they were gradually less able to cope with infection. As a result, they would develop AIDS, and die. For a short while, the Western media was full of images of dying babies, and the outpouring of charitable aid was enormous. However, interest gradually waned, and by the end of the century it was generally assumed that the issue had been addressed. It had not.

In 1999, the White Rose Initiative (WRI) was contacted by the new Director of Hospitals in Sighisoara – Dr Cornell Puskas. During an initial tour of his five hospitals, he was taken to the paediatric hospital, to a ward with 16 abandoned children, all tied into their cots. The children were aged between 9 months and 12 years old, and all awaited transfer to children's mental hospitals, where – thankfully – there were no vacancies. The children stared vacantly at nothing; they rocked gently and made hardly a sound. It was impossible to tell which children had been born with brain damage, and which were merely the product of their abusive environment.

DOI: 10.4324/9781003255444-33

Puskas was reminded of a series of experiments with baby monkeys reared in isolation by Harlow, an American psychologist, which had concluded that no play creates a socially disturbed monkey (Suomi & Harlow, 1971). If otherwise isolated infant monkeys were given time in a playroom with normally developing monkeys, they grew up to be relatively normal. Puskas felt the parallels between the life experience of these 16 children and Harlow's isolate-reared monkeys were obvious. He set aside a playroom, and WRI employed a Romanian play-worker, named Edit Bus, to play with the children.

Edit reported additional deprivations: the children were not being fed properly; they were not bathed regularly; their nappies were changed no more than once a day; their ward was not kept clean; they had no sheets on their mattresses; and when they were ill, they were treated with shared needles. This was particularly shocking because some of them were believed to be HIV+. Their development was stunted in every way – the most extreme example being a ten-year-old boy who had the muscular-skeletal structure of a four year old.

Within the group of children there was a nine-month-old toddler, who was developing relatively normally. This was a stroke of good fortune for the project, as he unwittingly became our equivalent of Harlow's 'therapist monkey' – our 'therapist toddler'. In other words, his presence in the group clearly enabled some of the children to go back to the beginning and start their development again.

After a short time, Edit was joined by a playwork student from the UK – Sophie Webb. Sophie was completing the professional practice element of her playwork degree course. An extract from Sophie's reflective diary, written after her first day with the children, gives a powerful insight into her experience of joining the project.

These were my first impressions of the conditions at the hospital and the way the children are treated:

The silence. Every room was full of children in cots, but it was so quiet. Even when we entered the room there was no sound from the children. They just looked at us. The smell of urine in every room was almost unbearable.

The emptiness. Each room had just the cots with plastic mattresses. The children were dirty and wearing clothes that were too big for them. Some were wearing jumpers as trousers, and none of them were wearing shoes. There were rags around their waists, which I later found out were ripped up sheets, tied to keep the nappies in place. These rags were also used to tie the children to the cots. Most children were sitting rocking and others were standing up banging the sides of their cots against the walls. Giving the children a cuddle was strange as they either held on too tightly, or they remained stiff and unfeeling.

When I observed the children in the playroom, they were unaware of each other, fixed on their own activities – barely communicating. Some just sat and seemed bewildered and vacant.

Webb and Brown (2003)

It is hard to imagine a more disadvantaged and routinely abused group of children outside of a war zone. Yet despite all that, in the ensuing year every child was able to make remarkable progress – even those who had clearly been born with some form of identifiable brain damage.

Initially our approach was to work with individual children in the playroom, while the rest of the group explored their new environment. For example, among other specialised techniques, we used 'joining' and 'rhythm' to communicate and stimulate human connection.

Joining

The Option Institute's (2022) technique of 'joining' is similar to the playwork approach of working to each child's agenda. Option's approach accepts that autistic children are keen to form human relationships but cannot find a way that non-autistic people can understand. They also accept that autistic children want to play, but their play is difficult for us to recognize. In order to make a social connection we need to 'join' the child in their play, no matter how strange that play might be. When someone shows interest in their play, the child will return that interest. This leads to genuine human engagement, which in turn enables us to help the child learn and develop (Kaufman, 2014). We made good use of this approach during our time working in Sighisoara Paediatric Hospital. Sophie Webb's diary details the results.

We were keen to help a ten-year-old boy (mentioned previously) to walk independently, but he was frightened to do so. However, when Sophie 'joined' him in his favourite activity (obsessively playing with shoes), her relationship with him changed, and that gave him the confidence to take a risk.

NICOLAE

I made sure I spent some time with Nicolae today. I have played 'shoes' with him for the past two weeks and that appears to have led him to trust me. Today, after playing 'shoes' yet again, I stood him in the middle of the room, about four steps away from me. Usually he just sits down, but this time he walked towards me with his arms stretched out for a hug. I think these may have been his first independent steps (after ten years!).

Webb (2014, Day 18)

One four-year-old girl resisted social interaction of any kind. However, Sophie noticed that Elena looked extremely happy when standing in a corner by herself rocking and repeating the same sound over and over.

ELENA

Today I started to repeat the noises that Elena makes "waaaaoooo waaaaoooo" and her reaction was amazing! The look on her face was just like someone had spoken her language. It felt like a little breakthrough as you can rarely communicate with her. Touch is so important to her. I started to repeat this noise back to her and she responded by instigating the sequence when she saw me, exploring my face and trying to decide where the noise was coming from. By making myself the play environment, Elena was comfortable to allow herself the freedom to communicate and investigate.

Webb (2014, Day 29)

Rhythm

Trevarthen (1996), Davy (2008), and Sladen (2012) all suggest newborns come into the world with an understanding of the concept of rhythm. Indeed, it is one of the most fundamental developmental building blocks, and babies use their understanding of rhythm to interpret social relationships. In the following story, it was important to view Liliana as a little girl with the potential to learn and develop during her play, rather than as a child with a visual impairment. By using the simple device of a rhythmical song, it was possible to form a relationship very quickly and help a troubled child feel secure.

LILIANA

On my final day I came upon a very agitated four-year-old girl who had been left in a ward totally alone. She stood at the bars of her cot rocking back and forth, making strange hooting noises. Every so often she walked rapidly round the cot, before settling back into her rocking.

Her doctors said she was "blind and mentally retarded". I felt uncomfortable with this diagnosis, as she was clearly aware of my presence, and appeared to be reacting to my movements (albeit not in a very positive fashion). There was obviously something wrong with her eyesight, but a quick experiment with moving lights showed she had some level of residual vision – seeing shadows, at the very least. An added complication was her fear of men's voices. This was confirmed when I called her name, "Liliana". Straight away she retreated to the back of the cot.

The playworkers were wondering how they could work with her. How could they get beyond the obstacle of her poor sight?

I started singing to Liliana quietly: "Twinkle, Twinkle, Little Star". She calmed down immediately, moving her head to locate the sound. At the end of the song she made a noise in the back of her throat, which I interpreted as a request to sing again – a kind of play cue. I did this three times, and each time she moved closer to the sound.

Then I started to clap gently in time to the rhythm of the song. When I stopped, she reached for my hands and put them together – another cue for me to sing. I repeated the song three more times, and each time she gave the same cue. On the last occasion she not only took my hands, but also started clapping them together in time to the song. Finally, she picked up the rhythm of the song in her own hand movements and clapped in time to my singing.

This whole sequence took no more than five minutes. In that short space of time I was able to show the Romanian playworkers how to start making a relationship with Liliana by using rhythm and music.

Later that afternoon I went back into her ward, to find her rocking and hooting again. I called her name, "Liliana". She came across the cot, and felt for my hands. Clasping them together in hers, she started to clap our hands together in a rhythm that I recognized – "Twinkle, Twinkle, Little Star". This was truly a magic moment.

Brown (2014)

The power of group interactive play

Examples such as these demonstrate the ways in which specific techniques can help troubled children to move forward. However, the most powerful influence on the development of these 16 children was finding themselves in an environment that enabled them to interact with each other. Indeed, some of the children made degrees of developmental progress that none of us expected. They rapidly moved through Jennings' (2011) stages of development, as though they just needed to make one good connection with a stage before moving on rapidly towards the stage that might be considered appropriate to their particular age. The more able children were observed engaging in complex and abstract forms of symbolic play within four months of entering the therapeutic playwork project. According to Piaget (1951) symbolic play takes between two and three years to develop, and abstract cognition appears towards the end of that period. How was it that these children made such striking progress in such a short period of time?

Two observers collected research data independently using a combination of participant and rotating non-participant observation. To analyse the findings we used a derivation of a system originally designed to assess children's use of playgrounds (Brown, 2000). This analysis demonstrated that in the space of just six months, the children showed strong improvement in their social interaction skills, their motor skills, and their general enjoyment of life. All children showed some progress in the following developmental categories: freedom of action, flexibility, cognitive interaction, self-discovery, creativity, and problem solving. Perhaps unsurprisingly, the one area where the findings were more mixed was the development – or otherwise – of emotional equilibrium. Overall, the developmental changes observed were substantial, especially given the short timescale. How could such significant changes be explained?

Play is the answer.

Our observations showed that nothing remarkable changed in the lives of these children, other than their experience of the WRI project. Playworkers Edit and Sophie had to untie the children in the morning, bathe them, feed them properly, work with them in the playroom all day, and then take them back to the ward in the evening, where the nurses would tie them to their cots again. They would then receive no human attention until the playworkers arrived in the morning. So, it is possible to state that the changes in the children were a direct consequence of the therapeutic playwork project.

Clearly the children were now being treated with kindness and being fed properly by the playworkers. However, although that may account for the more relaxed mood of the children, it is unlikely their developmental steps were a direct result of those factors. On the contrary, we became convinced that interactive social play was the most significant factor in achieving change. In other words, the major catalyst in bringing about change was the playful environment we created, rather than any specific work undertaken with individual children. That is not to undervalue those techniques, but the strongest influence on the children's development was undoubtedly the children themselves. Their engagement with each other was a joy to behold and left no doubt in our minds that play had become what Drew and Nell (2021, p. 23) later described as the "safe context for constructing meaningful self-knowledge and revitalizing the human spirit" (Figure 27.1).

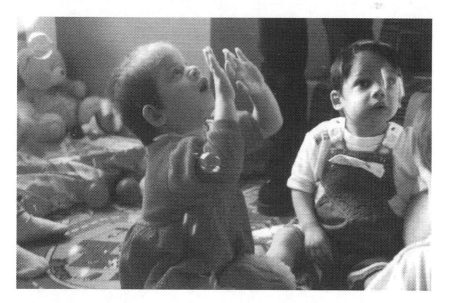

FIGURE 27.1 Bubbles.

References

Brown, F. (2000) Play Value Research Project. In *Proceedings of 2nd Theoretical Playwork Conference, 'New Playwork – New Thinking?'*, 21–22 March 2000. Ely: Play Education

Brown, F. (2014) *Play and playwork: 101 stories of children playing*. Maidenhead: Open University Press

Davy, A. (2008) Exploring rhythm in playwork. In F. Brown & C. Taylor (Eds.) *Foundations of playwork*. Maidenhead: Open University Press

Deletant, D. (1995) *Ceausescu and the securitate: Coercion and dissent in Romania, 1965–1989*. London: Hurst & Co. (Publishers) Ltd

Drew, W. & Nell, M. (2021) *Self active play awakens creativity, nurtures self discovery, inspires optimism*. Melbourne Beach, FL: Institute for Self Active Education

Gloviczki, P. (2004) Ceausescu's Children: The Process of Democratization and the Plight of Romania's Orphans. *Critique: A Worldwide Student Journal of Politics*. Fall, 2004, pp. 116–125. Illinois State University

Jennings, S. (2011) *Healthy attachments and neuro-dramatic play*. London: Jessica Kingsley Publishers

Kaufman, R. (2014) *Autism breakthrough: The ground-breaking method that has helped families all over the world*. London: Vermilion: London

Nelson, C., Fox, N. & Zeanah, C. (2014) *Romania's abandoned children: Deprivation, brain development and the struggle for recovery*. Cambridge, MA: Harvard University Press

Option Institute (2022) *Autism Treatment Center of America*. [Online] Available from: <https://option.org/about-us/autism-treatment-center-of-america/> [Accessed 14 August 2022]

Piaget, J. (1951) *Play, dreams and imitation in childhood*. London: Routledge and Kegan Paul

Sladen, D. (2012) Pediatric Auditory Assessment: Using Science to Guide Clinical Practice. In *22nd Annual Audiology Conference*, 16 February 2012, Rochester, MN: Mayo Clinic

Suomi, S. & Harlow, H. (1971) Monkeys without play. In J. Bruner, A. Jolly, & K. Sylva (Eds.) (1976) *Play: Its role in development and evolution*. Harmondsworth: Penguin Books

Trevarthen, C. (1996) How a Young Child Investigates People and Things: Why Play Helps Development. In *Keynote speech to TACTYC Conference 'A Celebration of Play'*, November 1996, London

Webb, S. (2014) Therapeutic playwork project: Extracts from a reflective diary. In F. Brown (Ed.) *Play and playwork: 101 stories of children playing*. Maidenhead: Open University Press

Webb, S. & Brown, F. (2003) Playwork in adversity: Working with abandoned children in Romania. In F. Brown (Ed.) *Playwork theory and practice*. Buckingham: Open University Press

28

PLAY AND THE PARADIGM SHIFT

*Barrington Powell – Practitioner in Therapeutic
and Specialised Play/Arts and Patient Experience*

The privileged position I find myself in as a practitioner of play within the hospital wards began in early 2001 when I became a Clown Doctor after responding to an advert in a newspaper. I met a wonderful chap called Colin Maher who was down to earth and looked like a young version of Sid James from the 'Carry On' movies. Colin seemed to bubble with an innocent mischief. He was the first Clown Doctor in the UK and was instrumental in helping set up the programme in Europe to provide laughter to sick children in hospitals on a regular basis.

It is important to note that my sister had spent most of her early life in and out of hospitals because of a congenital heart condition. As a sibling I knew the tedium of waiting around in long hospital corridors for my sister, the patient, to be poked, prodded or called into mysterious rooms as I stared blankly, at the cartoon characters painted on the walls. Those minutes of waiting would spiral into hours of boredom for a six year old. My sister is one of the strongest people I know and I am immensely proud of her, I'm not sure that she knows that the work I do has been inspired by her.

I eventually would give up my role as a Clown Doctor to run my own programmes in two separate hospitals. Orly's Magic was created with the love and support of two amazing people, the Feddys, who in memory of their daughter had created something beautiful after seeing me work in 2012.

The below stories are taken from this period.

CASE STUDIES

1: General admissions: A traditional open ward with a number of bays

We begin on a general assessment ward, which as the name suggests means patients are assessed on this ward so a diagnosis can be given and the patient

DOI: 10.4324/9781003255444-34

can then be referred to a specialised ward that can provide treatment for their specific condition.

When I began working on this chapter I was contacted by my Agent who informed me that a past patient was trying to contact me. I realised the words she had sent were extremely powerful because they were authentic. With Ms Hannah Hodgson's permission, I have included that conversation below:

> Hello, please can you put me in touch with Barrington at some point today?
>
> This is quite a long story but stick with me! In 2015 I was in the Children's Hospital for 6 months back in 2015. Barrington came in weekly and was such a light for both my mother and I during that time. While I was an inpatient, I won my first ever poetry competition. Both Barrington and the play leader Dave made the day special for me. Barrington did an amazing picture, framing (my poem for me). I'm now a freelance poet and my first full length collection is coming out in February. I want to include that poem and if possible the picture Barrington made for me. To do this I need his written permission. Could you put us in touch? The deadline is looming (today), and his contact info hasn't been very easy to find.
>
> Thanks for your time.
>
> Best wishes,
> Hannah

It goes without saying that I am immensely proud of Hannah's achievements with finding a professional publisher to showcase her talents. Dave is one of the best play specialists I have had the pleasure of working alongside.

Dave had told me that Hannah had won a competition and asked me if I could illustrate a picture around the poem for her and then frame it and make the day extra special, which we did, and then we both surprised her with it. Dave always went the extra mile for his patients. That evening I drew the picture. The poem was about the plight of the refugee crisis, and Hannah's words were extremely powerful and beautiful. We presented the framed poem to her the following day. I had not realised how much of an impression this had made on Hannah but when asking to include it in her own book, she mentioned the impact it had. In her own words she said it had provided light to her in a dark time. "I remember a time in particular when I was moved into the side room and both you and Dave came and sat down, and we just talked. I really needed that".

Sometimes it can be the simplest acts of kindness which make the biggest difference. A simple conversation is sometimes all it takes.

Many a time Dave would be the catalyst for me to create what would appear to be random acts of chaos, simply to make one another laugh for the amusement of the patient. On one occasion I took to sticking a surgical glove over the top of my head so that I could become a chicken (I had heard the real Patch Adams used to do this). Both the patient and Dave creased up.

Dave would simply shake his head in despair along with the patient in agreed unison that I was simply off my head, but suddenly the patient who may have been quiet for days was coming out of their shell and had forgotten their problems and had entered another world; and before you knew it they were talking with Dave in absolute agreement and looking forward to the following week's visit. I cannot tell you how beautiful these moments are.

2: Renal dialysis: An enclosed ward containing 4/5 machines with chairs and a side room containing 1 machine or bed

Here the work is completely different from a standard ward visit. The children would be attached to their machines receiving treatment for at least three times a week for over four hours. Many are waiting for the possibility of a transplant. Mums and dads would be by their sides, trying to juggle a work balance with their child's condition, whilst trying to sort out a family unit which may also have siblings to consider. Sp, the work is not just about life-saving medication for the patient but the dynamics that it has upon a family unit. Tied up in all of this are stress, guilt, frustration and anger, and feelings of utter helplessness. It is not just one patient you are dealing with, but the forgotten siblings and parents who also need a virtual hug.

When I first visited this type of ward I saw parents looking downbeat and exhausted. The four or five beds (which included a side room) became the answer. This was a community of characters brought together under exceptional but 'shared' circumstances. There would be morning dialysis and afternoon dialysis for a different set of patients all in need of those life-saving machines. I had been asked to visit as part of my ward rounds, a different approach was needed because you had young patients and older patients and different cultures and yet all with that 'shared' experience of three times a week attending the same room, and somehow I was on an unknown mission to create a small community within that ward.

This set-up is similar to those set up by the Welcome Trust where clinical trials for specific conditions would take place. This had a set of children arriving from far away to receive treatment on the same ward, week upon week. Imagine having to travel from Ireland or Scotland to receive the only specialised treatment to make a difference to your child; families unable to up sticks because of work commitments or extended family responsibilities. Then you start to realise the unbelievable stories the patients go through, and with this understanding you realise there are numerous factors at play here and to have something other than treatment to focus on makes a real difference. The patient comes in happier, which then makes the nursing staff's job easier, and you become an extended family community complete with a hidden support network taking care of the emotional needs of people rather than just the physical/medical needs.

There was an incredible playworker there called Emma who was devoted to the children. Her position was funded privately by the Welcome Trust who knew the importance this would have on the patients' well-being, and she was an intricate part of the team.

'Children in Need' captured one of my visits whilst on these wards. On entering Renal Dialysis a young boy of about the age of three shouted out my name with so much love and affection because he was so excited to see me. It beats any Oscar you could ever win. Another patient squeaked a nurse's nose. We all created a camaraderie through those weekly regular visits which started to have a huge impact on everyone present.

It became a proper club, and just like my days working at Pontins, we would play Hoy Bingo. I had not realised my early days of working in the holiday camp environment running a children's club would be so important. Hoy Bingo was a card game I had learnt in my days as a Blue Coat, in which we would call out a series of playing cards. We had suddenly turned the whole Renal Dialysis Unit into a gambling den! AND everyone loved it! I would snaffle up a prize from the play cupboard (signed for obviously) but it did not matter if the prize was good, bad or rubbish; quite frankly the worse the gift, the better, because it was never about the present it was about the joy of all being together. The staff would join in and it was a golden time.

Genuine bonds of respect, which never over-stepped the line of professionalism, were unknowingly being forged. In the words of a mum and with her kind permission I shall let her tell the story:

My son was on home dialysis until he caught a really bad infection which meant that he had to start hospital dialysis at the age of 2.

This meant we had to travel to Manchester from Burnley sometimes 5 times a week for treatment and my son would have to sit on a bed or a chair for 4 hours at a time. As you can imagine trying to keep a child entertained whilst hooked up to a machine is extremely difficult. The only thing he could look forward to was Barrington Powell coming to entertain him with his magic balloons and making general silliness. My sons face lit up every time he was around and it helped to take my sons mind off the tough treatment he was having. It also helped me as a parent as it cheered me up no end and helped put a smile on everyone's' faces and helped us to forget for an hour or so the tough times we were having. The importance of play within a hospital setting helps the children forget their troubles and makes them feel like a normal child if only for a while.

3: Oncology: A mixture of open bays and cubicles for isolation as well as standard cubicles

No other word can manifest the same fear and dread, as the word 'cancer'. I have seen how it is able to take lives and cause more suffering than any other disease. It has the ability to offer false hope and will try and rob you of your dignity, and yet somehow I have also seen bravery like no other and beautiful moments of humanity through stories that continue to inspire, some of sorrow and some of joy. No child should ever go through this sort of treatment. It is a word no child should ever hear and yet some do.

I hate cancer.

The below story is given with kind permission of Milly's mum who is not only a parent, but is a nurse also and runs a beautiful charity called 'Milly's Smiles'.

I walk into a ward and there is a newly admitted patient who would later be known as the Milsters. Dad is sitting in the corner and Milly is propped up on her bed and on her table amongst a collection of books and felt tip pens is a chess board. I used to love chess and haven't played for ages! I was quite good if I recall and so was up for a game and so was Milly. Milly's dad watched smiling as Rook took Bishop. At first I was going to let Milly win but as the game continued, I started to get into it. Dad just continued smiling! Suddenly I saw a chance and my Bishop took Milly's Queen. I was going to win this easily. But try as I might I could not! Milly without her central piece continued to make counter move and dodge check mate. Eventually it was obvious no one was going to win. It was stalemate fair and square! Quite frankly I was exhausted. Dad was beaming with pride and with a lilt of Blackburn dialect in his accent, said the words I will never forget. "She's really good isn't she, especially considering she has only been playing for a week!"

I had total respect for Milly that week and always had from that day on. She still inspires me to this day.

A few weeks later I got a call from an Agent, asking me if I had a cowboy outfit for one of their prestigious clients. I had, but I hadn't realised when I accepted the booking that it was for a Line Dancing Cowboy Instructor! This would be fine if not for one tiny problem which was that I have never done line dancing in my life. The booking meant I had to host a huge corporate function with over 100 professional adults for their top awards function, and at the end of their presentation I would have to perform a proper 'legitimate' line dance.

I think I held my head in my hands as I retold the story to Milsters that day!

"I have to dress up as a Cowboy and do a line dance!" I sounded like a man at the end of his tether!

"Oh that's ok" she responded, giving a knowing glance towards her mother. "Mum use to do LINE DANCING and I am sure she can teach you a dance. Isn't that right mum?"

Poor Lorraine looked traumatised. Milly beamed.

Next week the whole Bay and most of the Oncology Department had cowboy hats on as we did a song called the 'Watermelon Crawl' which Lorraine suggested I should do. That song is still on my mobile phone. Many of the Staff joined in, as did the children, some attached to their machines, and parents also strutted their stuff. After a number of those sessions, somewhat like a few bad episodes of 'Strictly Come Dancing', I managed to vaguely get the footsteps slightly coherent! One evening, somewhere in a swanky location in Blackpool, Milly helped me blag my gig and I hope I made her proud!

I will let Lorraine (Milly's Mum) continue the story in her own words:

I recall that initial meeting like it was yesterday. I was sat with my daughter Milly on her hospital bed, in a bay with 3 other children. All of a sudden chaos reigned. There was a lot of noise and suddenly this man dressed like a clown appeared in the room, and the room just lit up. For the next hour we were transported from parents who were petrified as to what the future held for their child, to being part of a highly entertaining performance.

Barrington performed magic, engaging every child and including them in his circle of fun. They laughed, they were enthralled by the magic tricks; we were drawn into a world of fun, frolics and fantasy. Balloons were modelled into the most amazing creations and there was one made for every child. No one was left out. Everyone, including parents were made to feel part of this fun world.

From this day on, Barrington became such an important part of Milly's and my life. We looked forward to his visits to the ward with so much excitement. We discovered that Barrington was not only a fabulous entertainer but he was a very talented artist. He drew a wonderful caricature of Milly, he incorporated everything about her in so much detail, and to this day this remains so very special to me. Nothing was every too much trouble, Barrington would go to the ends of the earth to make the children and the parents forget their troubles. He made so many people happy in what were very emotive circumstances.

Milly developed an interest in magic and Barrington thoroughly encouraged this. He bought her a magic set which she loved and helped her learn some tricks of the trade. He spent many hours with her during our time in the hospital, and became very special to us,

Milly loved him to bits. We became privileged to learn about Barrington the person, not just the entertainer. He is a genuine warm, caring man who wears his heart on his sleeve. He would often regale us with tales from his life and have us in fits of laughter. I can honestly say that he made our whole experience in the hospital so much better – without him it would have been a different story.

Sadly, we lost Milly. Words can never explain the pain and sadness that have followed.

Barrington kept in touch, by now we regarded him as a very close friend and one whom we would be lost without. He made a beautiful balloon display of flowers for Milly's funeral, which she would have loved.

In 2015 I started up a charity in Milly's honour, called Milly's Smiles. We needed a logo and there was only one person for the job – Barrington. What an amazing logo he produced, we met up in a fish and chip shop one rainy Sunday afternoon and he spent hours coming up with different designs, nothing was too much trouble, he had the patience of a saint that afternoon.

Barrington will always have a special place in my heart, he made Milly's last year so much better. To hear her laugh and joke with him when she was going through so much will be something I will never forget. Every once in a while someone special comes into your life. Barrington is one of those people – truly remarkable with a heart of gold.

When Milly passed away it truly broke my heart. The bell had rung which meant treatment had been finished and all looked hopeful. All we have at times of sorrow is to hold onto our stories, and to share those precious memories, in the hope of making sense of life. Sometimes life is cruel. Sometimes situations are simply out of our hands. Try as we might, we cannot change or control the outcome.

At the same time as this story there was more sorrow of children who did not make it, but there was also a lot of happiness for children whose treatment had been successful, which left its own bitter sweet taste, of guilt and pain. Amongst the sadness there had been those happy memories to cling onto when sorrow would be too painful or would slowly subside. It never fully goes away but those memories make it bearable.

The work on this ward was moving and many tears were shed. You should not take your work home with you and you should remain as professional as you can. BUT, should it hurt? Too right it should, because if it ever stops hurting, then that for me would be the day to give up. We are all human and this Ward hurt, but we were all trying desperately to make a difference.

Milly's memory has created a charity that provides those essential items in the form of a bag, so as you arrive on the ward you get items that are a godsend and much needed. After Milly's funeral and a few days later I was asked if I could help design a logo for Milly and Lorraine's charity, it was an honour to do the logo and every time I see that bag, which is now in three major hospitals in the UK I feel very proud to have known Milly.

4: Music to Make Pizzas By! Volume 27

Emma (a teaching assistant) was making pizza with a patient that week. Every Friday there was a baking lesson which helped establish a weekly routine in the hospital for the children. It was important to have some sort of structure to the week so that the children realised what day of the week it was, and also for them to have something to focus on and more importantly to look forward to. I said I would help and also bring in some Italian music. A little patient had missed the Friday morning session and so we managed to be in a separate ward. This little patient was only six and he was very stern and extremely serious.

I was rather proud of my compilation of 'Music to Make Pizzas By! Volume 27'. It was the equivalent of a 1980s mix tape of Italian classics. I always sang every time I made Pizza with Emma and we would splat the dough on the table as I sang my own rendition of 'It's All About that Bass'. Occasionally I would step onto an unblown balloon and stretch it upwards and pluck it like the strings from a double bass whilst warbling the chorus. Emma would give me one of her wonderful withering looks which consisted of her rolling her eyes heaven bound and looking on in utter despair as she shook her head. As the flour was being sprinkled into the air this was my perfect opportunity to roll up my trousers and wrap myself into a cubicle curtain and pretend that I was a lady singing along to a song called 'Bella Bella Signorina ...' as I unfurled from the curtain, I swirled with a bit too much gusto and went flying straight into a pirouette that sent me somersaulting towards the floor! The last thing I recall was Emma and my little friend's mouth agog! SPLAT – I genuinely hit the deck. Emma tried not to laugh but could not control herself and was helpless with laughter, my little friend looked at her, looked at me, tried to look stern and then looked back at Emma and before you knew it he had also cracked up. It was as if Emma had given him permission to lighten up. It was the most magical thing you could see and hear.

Through the following weeks this little chap started to laugh more and open up to both of us. Emma was once again giving a lesson and I was quite clearly getting into the teaching session far too much, that our little pal gave me a bewildered look as if to say this stuff was far too easy for him and that I was quite clearly just ridiculous. Through the next couple of weeks he began to laugh but also with his now trade mark stern looks.

When I heard the news that the cancer was just too virulent and nothing could be done for him, it was crushing, but you have to remain as professional as you can because you still have other children to see and have to make everyone happy.

It was time to say goodbye and again it would be one of the hardest things I would have to do. I have done it before and it is not nice, but you feel honoured that you made such a difference. The teachers had already been in and had prepared me.

There's a room you realise at the end of the corridor where you know it is time to pay your respects and to say farewell. Life continues but you are just aware that here there is dignity, solemnity and private respect in this part of the hospital which is unspoken.

Emma and Alex were there to help me, by the door and at my side as I was to enter the room. They had warned me that it could be less than a few hours that he had left, and I cannot thank them both enough for being there for me that day. He won't be able to say much and he is very much out of it, they had said. I thanked them and slowly opened the door and crept into the room like treading onto a carpet full of eggshells.

I was aware that he may be sleeping or in some form of discomfort and sedated, that he might not be able to hear me. I whispered as quietly as I could a "Hello" followed by his name and the words "I just wanted to let you know I'm here", whilst in my head I was just wishing to say goodbye and to say a private prayer to anyone who would listen and then discreetly leave. As soon as he heard my voice, suddenly his eyes opened wide and he lit up, just like it was any normal day and he had been expecting me.

Of all the things to be happening in this situation I was not expecting this. In your head you are thinking, but you are meant to be dying, surely this is the wrong patient? You are trying to be as professional as you can and yet you cannot say any of the things you really want to say. I looked at him and managed to smile and luckily the words came, without over stepping the mark and I was able to tell my little friend what I needed to say "... You do know I care don't you?" I said it in a way to be truthful but not to cause distress and to be as genuine and sincere as I could and then he did the most remarkable thing I have ever witnessed. He looked straight into my eyes and said "Of course I do ..." and without missing a beat he did one of his frowns and said, "Now get on and make that balloon. I want a motorbike!"

I made the balloon, which takes five balloons and a bit of time to make and I accidentally let go of one balloon and he laughed his head off and told me off which he always did, and I eventually presented him with the balloon and said goodbye as I would normally do as if it had been a routine visit. That was the morning just before noon and after lunch I had been told he had passed away.

It has been almost 25 years since I first stepped onto the hospital wards. Since then I have done over 4,000 hospital visits. There will always be stories which are heartbreaking but there are also tales of joy. In a world that can often be cruel, I am so grateful to be able to do this wonderful job, which has become a vocation rather than work. I finish as I started, which is to simply say that these stories are some of the most precious gifts I have and that they are worth more to me than any material wealth that you could possess and more importantly that no child is ever forgotten.

Reference

Milly's Smiles – https://www.millyssmiles.org/

29

PLAYING BEYOND THE BOUNDARIES

How the role of the Health Play Specialist can benefit adults in healthcare

Irene O'Donnell – NHS Hospital Trust lead for therapeutic play, recreation, and youth services

Play is fun, relaxing, and calming. It encourages children and young people (CYP) to be curious and make sense of the world they live in. Through play CYP can understand complex situations, improve communication skills, and reduce stress and anxiety.

Children learn through play, explore their emotions and feelings, and learn to take risks, while enabling children to learn to fail and master new skills. Play is a fundamental right of every child according to the United Nations Convention on the Rights of the Child (UNCRC), stating that "Every child has the right to play and access to recreation" (UNICEF, 1991). Play can also be viewed as a catalyst for learning, expression of oneself, for pleasure or for purpose or non-purposeful reasons.

Play can improve your health and well-being. When experiencing fun and joy your brain releases more of the feel-good hormone dopamine, which has been linked to increased memory, creativity, and positive mental health (LEGO, 2018). Play can improve your mood, increase energy levels, bring feelings of relaxation and pleasure, and is linked to better health outcomes (Play England, 2022). Maintaining optimal levels of well-being is crucial for increasing the best chances of having a good quality of life (NHS, 2022). The benefits of play for children are widely accepted, but these benefits can span across all generations bringing joy, pleasure, and a sense of connection (Whitaker & Tonkin, 2021).

The benefits of play for all ages

Play can be liberating and freeing for children, so with all the evidence and widely acknowledged benefits of play for our younger generation, can these benefits extend into adulthood? We do not lose our sense of fun or need for social interaction, enjoyment, and pleasure as we grow old. In fact, it is suggested that

DOI: 10.4324/9781003255444-35

the need for meaningful connection increases with age (Suragarn et al., 2021). Adults also need opportunities to master new skills and support life-long learning. So, could play still be a valuable resource for adults too?

According to Dr Stuart Brown (2010), founder of the National Institute of Play (USA), the beneficial effects of partaking in even small amounts of play can extend through our lives. Brown says play can make us more productive and happier in everything we do. The Lego foundation are avid ambassadors for play for all ages and are known for using the slogan '0-99' on Lego boxes and products. They state, "Play brings us together and increases trust within teams. It fosters an experimental mindset and releases stress" (Lego, 2018).

The direct link between play and well-being can be observed in the pleasure taken from engaging in an activity that brings joy. For some this may be playing physically such as exercise or team sports; for others partaking in mindful activities such as jigsaw puzzles, word searches, or sudoku bring feelings of enjoyment. Play can present opportunities through the creative arts such as singing, dancing, painting, or sculpting. Many people receive a sense of achievement from knitting, baking, or growing vegetables. A game of bingo can be hugely exciting and rewarding – especially if you win! Whatever the activity may be, the essential ingredients are interest, feel good emotions, fun and joy.

The transferable skills of a HPS into adult care

Health Play Specialists (HPSs) and Youth Support Coordinators (YSCs) are a vital part of the team in helping to care for CYP in healthcare (Faulconbridge et al., 2019). They provide preparation, distraction, and coping strategies which support medical and nursing staff to deliver treatments or investigations. Using play as a tool, HPSs help reduce anxiety surrounding healthcare procedures, thus increasing cooperation and engagement with treatments. HPSs have been historically trained to work with CYP up until their 18th birthday (NAHPS, 2022). However, I would argue the role of the HPS/YSC and their skills are substantially transferable to adults in healthcare, bringing similar positive benefits.

Play with young adults

The young adult population in healthcare is growing and so is the recognition that they have a unique set of needs being neither child nor adult (Healthy Teen Minds, 2022). Over recent years some healthcare organisations have started to provide bespoke care for young adults with the recognition that the brain does not finish developing until we reach around 25 (Mental Health Daily, 2022). Young adults can have similar needs to adolescents when using healthcare and therefore can greatly rely on the HPS or YSC to deliver this support. If the brain does not reach full development until we are around 25 years old, it is understandable that the young adult population may have needs in similar ways to those experienced in adolescence. Therefore, supporting the play and activity needs of young adults, especially when seeking healthcare, is vital.

Young adults having treatment for cancer have benefitted hugely from the support of YSCs funded by the Teenage Cancer Trust charity (TCT). Having cancer does not just affect you physically, but also impacts on your emotional well-being and mental health (TCT, 2022). Receiving support from a YSC to help manage emotions, engage in therapeutic play or activity, and experience social connection has been described as making a bad situation more bearable (TCT, 2022). YSCs provide social and emotional support during and after treatment and use play and activity therapeutically to provide connection, and a sense of normality in an otherwise very abnormal situation.

Play with adults with learning disabilities and Autism

Another group of adults that benefit from HPSs support are those with learning disabilities (LD) and Autism. For people with LD and/or Autism the hospital environment can be overwhelming and frightening (Whitaker & Tonkin, 2021). This can increase anxiety and difficulties with accessing timely healthcare. The Equality Act (2010) requires that all people can access healthcare and not be discriminated against due to disability. Information shared with people with LD and Autism (and their carers) needs to be appropriate and tailored to help them manage treatment and procedures and reduce anxiety. The need for clear accessible information is often something the HPS will provide to meet their communication needs. This can be through providing social stories or visual story maps and photos to prepare for a procedure or hospital visit. People with an LD or Autism have an increased risk of mental health problems including higher levels of anxiety (NHSEI, 2019), they may need bespoke support, preparation, and coping techniques for managing hospital visits, medical treatment, and invasive procedures. The HPS is skilled and well placed to provide this support and improve their hospital experience.

LD and Autism are mentioned repeatedly in the NHS LongTerm Plan. The aim is to improve peoples' health by enabling them to access appropriate healthcare and to raise awareness throughout NHS teams to provide the right support (NHS, 2020). The HPS is in an advantageous position to lead on this work and use transferable skills to empower colleagues to include play in supporting all people with LD and Autism attending healthcare settings. University College London Hospital (UCLH) NHS Trust recently completed a two-year charity funded trial of a HPS working in adult services with people with LD and Autism. Early results are showing this role has made a difference to many patients who would have otherwise not managed to receive their treatment and has helped to reduce anxiety and enhance patient experience for this group of adults. An example of this was a 40-year-old patient with an LD that needed an MRI scan but was very anxious. With support and preparation, he managed to cooperate and complete the scan without general anaesthetic (which was a risk factor for him).

Play with older people

For elderly people loneliness is identified as one of the biggest risks to their health and so supporting them in hospital through play and activities can be vital for their well-being (NHS, 2022). The HPS is well placed to use their skills throughout the age ranges, often being highly skilled communicators and enablers, they can support adults using similar techniques that they have used within paediatric settings. Distraction and coping strategies can be just as successfully used with adults as they are with the children. Who hasn't appreciated a staff member talking to them whilst having a blood test or procedure to take their mind off what is happening? Keeping someone calm, reassured, and able to tolerate the treatment or procedure is a beneficial skill enabling things to happen more smoothly, efficiently, avoiding delays and less likely to cause trauma or impact on the emotional health and well-being of the patients. Childhood experiences can impact on subsequent healthcare interactions and so adult patients may carry with them trauma from living with a long-term or chronic condition that they still need emotional and social support for (Tonkin, 2014).

Older people still have the need for social connection and activities that help them think, learn, and relax. People with dementia have been noted to greatly benefit from familiar activities such as bingo, craft activities, games, and puzzles. Playing with dolls can bring back positive memories of parenthood or childhood when other memories are starting to fade (Dementia UK, 2022). Play and activity can bring older adults' comfort and happiness. Having dancing or singing sessions brings chances for social interaction and joy. It can reduce anxiety, improve quality of life, and help to preserve language and speech (Whitaker & Tonkin, 2021). Many local nurseries or preschools have linked up with their local care homes to bring the children to visit and interact with the residents. The multiple benefits this can bring to the older people and the children and staff are heart-warming. This was documented in a Channel 4 television show called *Old People's Home for 4 Year Olds* (2017).

A COVID-19 PANDEMIC CASE STUDY FROM UCLH NHS FOUNDATION TRUST – EVERY CLOUD HAS A SILVER LINING

Irene O'Donnell Reg HPS, Chloe Davis Reg HPS, Deborah Edgington Reg HPS, Kim Robinson RCN

Following the outbreak of COVID-19 patients from the paediatric wards at UCLH were transferred to Great Ormond Street Children's Hospital (GOSH) to release beds for the increase in adult patients with Covid. Adult patients were admitted to the wards and cared for by the paediatric team. Naturally the paediatric staff experienced a range of emotions ranging from feeling scared, overwhelmed, worried, to learning new knowledge, courage and feeling proud of rising to the challenge and embracing the changes they were presented with at work. What unfolded was a unique relationship between the staff and the adult patients.

Using play as a tool HPS helped reduce anxiety surrounding healthcare and treatments for so many of the older adult patients. Nursing staff would also join the play sessions which benefitted their own well-being and helped calm down anxious patients who had no visitors due to the Covid situation.

The medical team witnessed the effect play specialists had on their adult patients when they introduced to the wards a variety of quizzes, word games, bingo, and painting into the day-to-day care. The medical team have documented what they witnessed in an article which was published in 2021 (Lynn et al., 2020). The abstract reads:

It is recognised that delirium is common among older adult inpatients and correlated with negative outcomes. The gold standard care for delirium management is achieved using multicomponent interventions. Which components work best is not yet well defined. During the COVID-19 outbreak, a paediatric ward was repurposed to treat adult patients. Paediatric nurses and play specialists remained on the ward. It was observed that the paediatric ward aesthetic and the team's dedicated approach to cognitive stimulation and sleep promotion improved well-being among older adult patients. We propose that elements of paediatric care, primarily deployment of a play specialist, could be incorporated into a multicomponent intervention for delirium prevention and management.

Lynn et al. (2020)

Our team of play specialists and nursing staff were delighted that the benefits of play and the transferable skills of the HPS were successfully translated into adult care. Therapeutic play truly does make a difference to a patient's day, it has a positive mood enhancing effect on patients, brings joy and pleasure to often difficult situations and has a positive impact on our health and well-being. The COVID-19 crisis unwittingly provided a window into the world of play specialists and paediatric care – that is the 'silver lining'.

Play has multiple benefits across the lifespan that are certainly not exclusive to CYP. Adults who partake in regular play have been reported to have an increased sense of well-being which has a positive impact on physical and mental health (Brown, 2010). Play can take all forms and ranges from physical, creative, or learning activities to non–purposeful activities for pleasure. Play has unique benefits for different age groups but can also present similar benefits proven in paediatric settings. Those with different needs and abilities can benefit from having support from a HPS to help them manage anxiety around hospital and treatment, and play is a useful tool to enable this to happen (Figures 29.1 and 29.2).

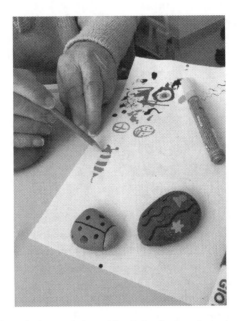

FIGURE 29.1 Pebble painting activity with adults during their time on the paediatric wards at UCLH during COVID-19, April 2020.

(Credit Chloe Davis)

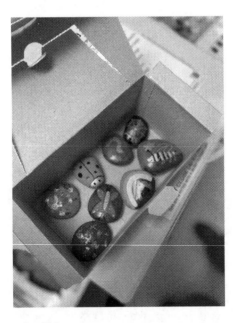

FIGURE 29.2 Decorated pebbles.

(Credit Chloe Davis)

The HPS is a skilled practitioner who has so much transferable knowledge and skills which bring value and benefits to adults throughout their lifespan in healthcare. The future presents opportunities to expand and build on the role of the HPS to regularly work in adult healthcare settings and improve the experience of many people within healthcare services. One day soon it could be possible to provide play for all ages in healthcare – a real silver lining!

> We don't stop playing because we grow old; we grow old because we stop playing
>
> *George Bernard Shaw*

References

Brown, S. (2010) *Play: How It Shapes the Brain, Opens the Imagination, and Invigorates the Soul.* Harmondsworth: Penguin

Dementia UK (2022) *Using Dolls in Dementia Care (Doll Therapy).* [Online] Available from: < https://www.dementiauk.org/get-support/living-with-dementia/doll-therapy/> [Accessed 4 August 2022]

Equality Act 2010 (c.15). [Online] Available from: <https://www.legislation.gov.uk/ukpga/2010/15/contents> [Accessed 11 July 2022]

Faulconbridge, J., Hunt, K. & Laffan, A. eds. (2019) *Improving the Psychological Wellbeing of Children and Young People.* London: Jessica Kingsley Publishers

Healthy Teen Minds (2022) *Young People and Young People's Organisations* [Online] Available from: <https://healthyteenminds.com/youngpeople/> [Accessed 22 December 2022]

LEGO (2018) *LEGO Play Well Report 2018.* [Online] Available from: <https://www.ncbi.nlm.nih.gov/pmc/articles/PMC2475802/> [Accessed 10 July 2022]

Lynn, M., Goulden, B., Parma, M., Knopp, P., Yeung, M., Giles, I., Davies, C., Espinosa, A. & Davis, D. (2020) *Play Attention! Therapeutic Aspects to Play in Delerium Prevention and Management.* [Online] Available from: <https://pubmed.ncbi.nlm.nih.gov/33364438/> [Accessed 10 July 2022]

Mental Health Daily (2022) *At What Age Is The Brain Fully Developed?* [Online] Available from: <https://mentalhealthdaily.com/2015/02/18/at-what-age-is-the-brain-fully-developed/> [Accessed 10 July 2022]

NAHPS (2022) *National Association of Health Play Specialists.* [Online] Available from: <https://www.nahps.org.uk/>training/ [Accessed 22 December 2022]

NHS (2019) *The NHS Long Term Plan* [Online] Available from: <https://www.longtermplan.nhs.uk/>[Accessed 22 December 2022]

NHS (2022) *Loneliness in Older People.* [Online] Available from: <https://www.nhs.uk/mental-health/feelings-symptoms-behaviours/feelings-and-symptoms/loneliness-in-older-people/> [Accessed 10 July 2022]

NHSEI (2019) *People with a Learning Disability Autism or Both: Liaison and Diversion Managers and Practitioner Resources.* [Online] Available from: <https://www.england.nhs.uk/wp-content/uploads/2020/01/Learning-disability-and-autism.pdf> [Accessed 10 July 2022]

Old People's Home for 4 Year Olds (2017) Channel 4 TV. 25 July 2017

Play England (2022) *All to Play for: Building Play Opportunities for All Children.* [Online] Available from: <https://www.playengland.org.uk/> [Accessed 5 August 2022]

Suragarn, U., Hain, D. & Pfaff, G. (2021) Approaches to Enhance Social Connection in Older Adults: An Integrative Review of Literature. *Aging and Health Research.* Vol. 1 (3) pp. 1–9 [Online] Available from: <https://www.sciencedirect.com/science/article/pii/S2667032121000275> [Accessed 10 July 2022]

TCT (2022) *Dealing with Cancer Emotionally.* Teenage Cancer Trust. [Online] Available from: <https://www.teenagecancertrust.org/information-about-cancer/dealing-cancer-emotionally> [Accessed 11 July 2022]

Tonkin, A. (ed) (2014) *Play in Healthcare: Using Play to Promote Child Development and Wellbeing.* Abingdon: Routledge

UNICEF (1991) *United Nations Convention on the Rights of the Child.* Svenska: UNICEF Kommitten

Whitaker, J. & Tonkin, A. (2021) *Play for Health Across the Lifespan: Stories from the Seven Ages of Play.* Abingdon: Routledge

30

PLAY WITH PURPOSE

The therapeutic value of play for
siblings of paediatric patients

Cala Hefferan – Certified Child Life Specialist

*Mikaela Sullivan – Certified Child Life Specialist
and Certified Therapeutic Recreation Specialist*

Siblings play a unique role within the family when a paediatric patient is diagnosed with an acute or chronic medical need. Siblings grow up often spending more time together than with other people in their family or community. Acknowledging the complexities of sibling relationships when an acute or chronic medical need arises is crucial. Family systems theory acknowledges that changes to one family member intrinsically affect the other members (Turner, 2018). Therefore, it can be understood that when considering the hospitalisation or diagnosis of chronic illness of one child, siblings have the potential to be significantly impacted. Structural and relational dynamics experienced by the siblings may include changes in proximity, communication, expectations, feelings of guilt, loneliness, and confusion (Deavin, Greasley, & Dixon, 2018; Gursky, 2007). Furthermore, siblings often find themselves unintentionally misunderstood and overlooked by caregivers (Levick et al., 2010; Deavin et al., 2018). The complex internal struggle of siblings to balance their emotional responses and needs with those of the patient and family can feel overwhelming. Research and our clinical experiences suggest that siblings often adapt their behaviours to sustain and balance the patient and caregivers' new emotional and physical demands (Deavin et al., 2018).

A new diagnosis or acute medical event within a family structure can threaten siblings' sense of security, health, and belonging, all basic needs that foundationally support milestone development. When faced with the ambiguous loss of a patient's health crisis, siblings' ability to process, grieve, and find meaning is significantly impacted; especially when they are unable to be involved, or their coping needs have not been identified or intervened upon (Boss & Couden, 2002). As child life professionals, we must ask ourselves, who's looking out for the needs of the siblings during stressful and traumatic times? Parents have a significant role in shaping the family dynamics to adapt to change. Though siblings may

DOI: 10.4324/9781003255444-36

not be physically present during diagnosis or treatment, they occupy an essential supportive role in the function of the family (Seymour, 2018). This change, for most children, is challenging to conceptualise because it is not always physical or concrete, and is highly likely not to reach closure. Family-stress perspective explains that we, as humans, have the motivation and capacity to cope with stressful events. However, the challenge lies when ambiguity blocks understanding and the ability to move forward (Boss & Couden, 2002).

The goal of interventions to counter the uncertainty of ambiguous loss is to help siblings build skills to live well with the stress and ultimately come to a better understanding of their situation and its impact on the patient and family. For siblings in the medical setting, play can provide such therapeutic value. Child life professionals are equipped with the skills needed to assess and mediate the siblings' stress response through play experiences including but not limited to play interactions aimed at promoting normalcy, increasing mastery, and ability to express and process emotions (American Academy of Pediatrics, 2021; Woodburn, Munn, Jones, Hoskins, Gill, Fraser, Dunbar, Duplechain, Boles, & Bennett, 2020).

Play for normalcy

Play provides siblings in the medical setting with something familiar. It gives them a sense of comfort to demonstrate their current developmental milestones in a new setting. Opportunities for play in the medical environment often lead to increased adjustment, confidence, and ability to adapt to the new environment and potential stressors. Play led by a child life professional builds rapport and empowers siblings with a sense of control. For some siblings, anticipatory anxiety leading up to a visit to the hospital can be overwhelming. Play interventions can provide an alternate focus and afford the siblings time to reappraise the situation and transition to the hospital environment. Similarly, play can provide siblings with an opportunity for socialisation with peers and other children experiencing similar situations. During play interactions, especially those led by the child, a child life professional can assess the siblings' developmental needs, identify hesitancies, and build rapport between the sibling and their caregivers.

Early in my career I worked as a child life associate (CLA) in a playspace designed especially for siblings and patients. The playspace was carefully designed to support structured and unstructured play activities. I often referred to the playspace as a fishbowl because it had large windows to display an outdoor play area and healing garden across the street. The space itself was painted with earth tones and included organised activity choices for various ages. As a CLA, I was usually one of the first healthcare professionals siblings met. I quickly learned that my initial encounter was pivotal to the siblings' appraisal of the healthcare environment. Communicating safety, trust, and acceptance to siblings and their caregivers during our time together was crucial. When I think of these times as a CLA, I remember how quickly a new pair of pants would get holes from hours of crawling around with siblings on the floor playing trains, house, farm, and dinosaurs. I remember reading book after book to the hesitant toddler waiting for the mother/father to return. I remember the countless hours of glitter art activities and refilling paint trays as a sibling put the final touches on their ceramic art piece. Most importantly I remember how play transformed cries and hesitation to smiles as siblings, with time, began feeling a sense of routine and eventually anticipation for entering their special place in the hospital.

Cala's Reflection

Play for increased understanding

Child life professionals assess the developmental age and needs of the siblings while fostering a safe environment in which the sibling can gain knowledge, express misconceptions, and ask questions.

The common goals of facilitated play interventions are:

- Preparation
- Clarifying misconceptions
- Familiarisation with medical equipment
- Gaining mastery

Preparation

Preparation aims to provide siblings with relevant and developmentally appropriate information to enhance their understanding and coping ability. Preparation decreases the siblings' response to stress (Gursky, 2007). When facilitating a play-based preparation, the child life specialist often considers how to prepare siblings for sensory input, including sights, sounds, smells, and how things may physically feel. Similarly, preparation activities may focus on siblings' understanding of a diagnosis and how it may impact the patient and family. Research supports that siblings prefer the advanced sharing of information related to the patient's disease because it builds understanding, reduces stress, promotes empathy, and strengthens coping (Burns-Nader & Hernandez-Reif, 2016; Deavin et al., 2018).

As a child life specialist in the paediatric intensive care unit, I would often meet siblings before they walked into the unit to visit the patient with their family. During my time with siblings, I would help them understand the physical space, and the changes they may observe in the patient's behaviour and health. Often using photos on my clinical iPad or a teaching doll with similar lines and tubes as the patient, I would allow siblings the opportunity to engage with the information before being exposed to it. All siblings' responses were met with an opportunity to learn more through age-appropriate language and opportunities to play. Examples of developmental responses could include:

Teens – quietly observing the function of machines, the necessity of lines and tubes, and the people in the room – following up with questions like, "When will the breathing tube come out?" or, "How many rounds of chemotherapy will my sister receive?"

School-age – using their fingers to engage and zoom on the iPad into every corner to see, "Where does that tube go?", and "Why is her hand wrapped like that?"

Toddlers – would point to the photo verbalising all the things they knew as it related to them, "Sissy!" and "That owie".

Mikaela's Reflection

When a child life professional builds a trusting therapeutic relationship on the foundation of psychological safety and age–appropriate information sharing, siblings are often willing to ask further questions to clarify their understanding.

Clarifying misconceptions

Play facilitated by a child life professional considers the developmental level, needs, and temperament of siblings. The siblings' developmental level will impact their cognitive understanding, the propensity for magical thinking, and feelings of jealousy or disconnect; all of which may lead to misconceptions about the patient's health and family dynamic.

A child life specialist can mediate sibling-led medical play to assess level of understanding, and interpret the gaps in siblings' knowledge of the information being shared or observed. Through play with a trusted facilitator siblings may reveal feelings of responsibility and their interpretation of medical treatment. When a child life specialist is present to assess and expand on siblings' understanding, siblings gain a greater sense of mastery over the ambiguous situation impacting their family and feel empowered to understand how the information does or does not relate to them (Figure 30.1).

I was consulted to meet with an eight-year-old patient with developmental delays and his three-year-old brother. Both patient and sibling were at a developmental level in which magical thinking was prevalent. The patient had a wound on his knee that was infected. Previously, under anaesthesia the wound had been cleaned and bandaged. The nurse needed to repack the sterile gauze and change the dressing. The patient and sibling were visibly upset, unable to regulate their behaviours, and non-compliance. I assessed these behaviours as fear and lack of understanding of the procedure and its importance. I designed the medical play bear (shown below) for the patient and sibling to address misconceptions. Under the teddy bear's bandage, I made a small incision similar to the patient's and filled it with red model magic and sterile gauze strips. I provided the patient and sibling with twee-zers, syringes, sterile gauze strips, and fresh bandages to manipulate, iden-tify, and discuss the patient's wound along with necessary needs. Through this play, the patient and sibling were able to attain accurate information and reappraise the situation as manageable.

Cala's Reflection

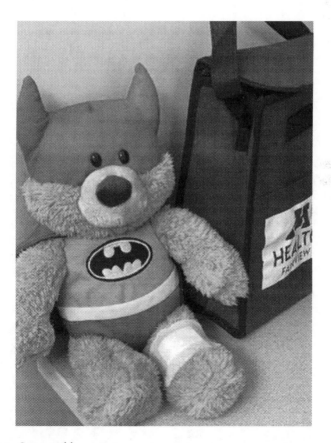

FIGURE 30.1 Super teddy.

Familiarisation with medical equipment

Presenting medical equipment through non-threatening exploratory play familiarises siblings with tangible items involved in the patient's care. Child life specialists often facilitate medical play using teaching dolls, toy doctor kits, stuffed animals with tubes and lines, and medical equipment such as ports, NG tubes, IV catheters, syringes, bandaids, and anaesthesia masks. Providing siblings with opportunities for directed and undirected medical play increases their sense of control, knowledge, and familiarity with the medical equipment and the environment (Figure 30.2). Additionally, research confirms that medical play allows siblings benefits similar to those that hospitalised children experience with child life intervention, i.e. reduction of anxiety, increased understanding, and demonstration of problem-solving skills (Burns-Nader & Hernandez-Rief, 2016; Gordon & Paisley, 2018).

This baby doll resulted from a sibling's independent medical play, unobserved, in the unit playroom. Can you predict what this child may have been observing in the hospital environment from the placement of these band-aids?

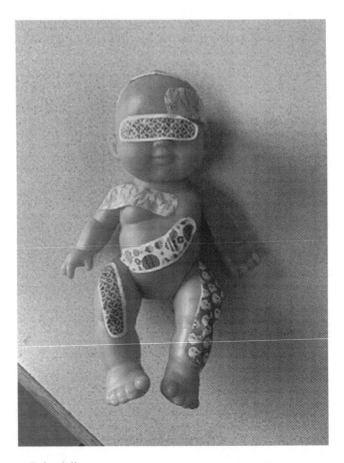

FIGURE 30.2 Baby doll.

Gaining mastery

During play, children process and appraise the experiences they perceive to have little control over and information that has been shared with them. Play is the platform in which siblings demonstrate mastery by exploring misconceptions, conquering fears, and developing confidence (Ginsburg, 2007). Child life specialists facilitate open-ended interventions in which siblings can practise the skills and concepts they understand and, in time, confidently demonstrate their knowledge. Gaining mastery is displayed by siblings in many different ways; appropriately manipulating medical equipment, sharing with a peer why the patient is in the hospital, or by showing their caregiver how to appropriately care for the patient's needs. Allowing siblings continued opportunities to demonstrate mastery can positively impact their ability to cope with the changes they are experiencing in their family and explore additional ways to process their emotions surrounding the situation (Figure 30.3).

Pictured above, three siblings following the discharge of a Neonatal Intensive Care Unit patient actively engaged in medical play with dolls that have g-tubes and familiar supplies. From the view of an adult, this photo demonstrates their age-appropriate understanding of the function and purpose of the g-tube and

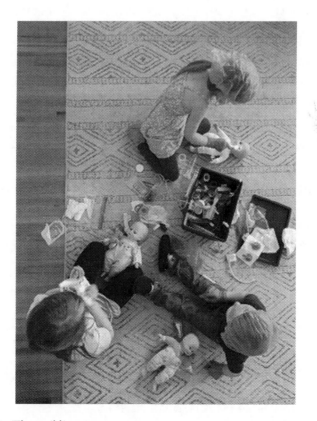

FIGURE 30.3 Three siblings.

how it is cared for in their home. It also reveals siblings' desire to manipulate supplies and understand how the patient's necessity for a g-tube impacts their family's life outside the hospital.

Play for processing, expression, and resiliency

When presented with the opportunity to play, some siblings gravitate towards a theme or specific toys they believe will help them articulate and tangibly manipulate misunderstood thoughts and emotions they are experiencing. As child life professionals, we have often observed themes unfold during play interactions with siblings in the hospital environment.

We have compiled the accompanying reflection outlining the evolution of processing, expression, and coping of a particular four-year-old sibling of a patient who has had a complex medical condition since birth. The patient and family have navigated an NICU admission, monthly ICU admissions, and transition to hospice care. Out of respect and confidentiality, names and personal details have been changed to protect the patient and family. We will call the sibling Noah.

> When Noah visited the hospital, it was often at the point in the patient's admission where there was no clear timeline for discharge, the family's routine was dismantled, as per his mother's statement, he was "needing a day with mom and (patient)". As a child life specialist who had built long-term trust and rapport with him, I was most often his first request, "Can we go to the big playroom together?" Noah would ask, referring to a room that was out of (the) patient's ICU room and off the unit. My answer would be, "Of course. What should we do when we get there?" His answer was always one of two things: Farm or Demo Derby. His play in the hospital rarely deviated.

Play is the medium through which siblings can safely express the worries and thoughts of their inner world. In addition, the repetition of habitual play can be soothing because the act engages the child's body in movement rather than stillness (Gaynard & Jessee, 2018). Unfortunately, siblings often silence their thoughts and emotions to protect their family, and the interpreted silence can be confusing for caregivers and lead to reciprocated silence. Because of this, siblings may have few opportunities to disclose their thoughts and the misunderstood emotions they are experiencing.

The opportunity to play with a child life professional can allow siblings to work through what is on their mind. In Noah's case, he sought this out immediately after entering the medical environment. He wanted to be close to his mother, yet he struggled to communicate his needs. While intended to protect each other, silence causes family members to become emotionally distant when they need each other the most (Deavin et al., 2018).

> On 'farm' day, we'd spend an hour lining up toy fences, plowing imaginary fields with combines and tractors in a particular sequence of events – depending on the made-up rain forecast. The crops would be harvested, they would be fed to the cattle, and then it was time to go back to planting crops. The cycle would continue until it was time to go back to the ICU. I had jobs directed by Noah, and he had tasks only reserved for him, like driving the combine.

Much like the need to normalise the hospital environment, children often feel the need for control through the ambiguous loss they are experiencing. This sense of control offers predictability, comfort, and knowledge, demonstrating mastery. For Noah, this was shown through his extensive knowledge of farming, coincidentally the career of his family members. It was a source of familiarity for him and a way for his skills to be acknowledged and validated.

Observing and engaging in child-directed play provides insight for the child life professional about how siblings are making sense of the healthcare environment and the needs of their brother or sister (Clark et al., 2018). During other hospitalisations, based on the acuity of the admission and what Noah had witnessed at home, there was a greater need for more expressive dynamics through play. Expressive play allows kids to symbolise aggressive and hostile feelings without fear of reprisal.

> When 'demo derby' was on the docket, Noah would spend a large portion of time lining up matchbox cars of all shapes and sizes around the pretend arena. There were some cars reserved ONLY for him. Noah's cars always appeared spectating in the front row of the derby. Others had to park in the back. Cars would be smashed and crashed, often requiring medical attention from first responders, played out by Noah. Then, right before they could be fixed, a ginormous monster truck would come barreling in, resulting in a head-on collision. These cars never seemed to catch a break, sometimes just like Noah.

As Camhi (2005, p. 214) shares, "Through play, children bring to life what overwhelms their mind". The action of the toys is a communication of thoughts being processed, just as words provide verbal processing for adults. For example, the child life professional may assess through play that siblings are struggling to put to words the confusion of separation, the ambiguity of loss, or insecurity during uncontrollable circumstances. Engaging siblings in expressive play provides a unique vantage point for identifying behaviours and expressing silenced and unresolved experiences and feelings.

> "Could my car watch from the front row today?" I would sometimes ask.
>
> "No, they shouldn't be seeing this. These cars are smashed", he would say.

Observing the themes of ambiguous loss, unclear injuries, and constant disruption demonstrated that Noah needed the opportunity to process his misconceptions and how they were impacting him. Perhaps Noah felt like the derby car being crushed by the monster truck with no prevail. The question for the child life professional while engaging and interpreting play is how can I identify and strengthen the siblings' ability to cope with adversity.

Masten (2014, p. 189) explains that coping is defined as "efforts to regulate the self or the environment under stress". Specifically, active coping, which builds resilience, includes problem-solving, seeking support, and accommodating strategies such as managing pain, alternate focus, and expressing stress and fears during adverse situations (Masten, 2014). Play interventions are aimed at helping children achieve mastery and a sense of agency, leading to expression and the motivation towards resilience. Child life professionals are uniquely trained and positioned to understand the language of siblings' play and provide opportunities to enjoy an alternate focus, rehearse coping strategies, and practise self-regulation (Woodburn et al., 2020).

> Engaging in cooperative play was not always agreed upon by Noah. We had to work on it. Together, I needed to understand the feelings of his (cars). While he needed to work on the feelings his cars/he was experiencing when the plotline of our play deviated, much like his life at home. Through his play, I watched Noah grow; in and out of the playroom. Able to articulate when he needed more information, identify his feelings through words and the language we used while together, and the ability to understand that he is safe to express his thoughts and feelings without fear of reprisal. It was bigger than Demo Derby day.

As literature, research, and our clinical reflections demonstrate, play, when facilitated or left thoughtfully unstructured, is an effective modality to express, process, and learn to cope with the ambiguity of a sibling's diagnosis or medical event. With the guidance of a child life professional, play has the potential to validate and diminish fears, bridge communication, and enable siblings to navigate questions and wonders that may otherwise be misunderstood or overlooked. Play with purpose empowers siblings to understand the complexity and uniqueness of their experience and move forward towards resilience.

References

American Academy of Pediatrics (2021) Policy statement: Child life services. *Pediatrics*, 147 (1).

Boss, P., & Couden, B. (2002) Ambiguous loss from chronic physical illness: Clinical interventions with individuals, couples and families. *Journal of Clinical Psychology*, 58 (11), pp. 1351–1360.

Burns-Nader, S., & Hernandez-Reif, M. (2016) Facilitating play for hospitalized children through child life services. *Children's Health Care*, 45 (1), pp. 1–21.

Camhi, C. (2005) Siblings of premature babies: Thinking about their experience. *International Journal of Infant Observation and Its Application*, 8 (3), pp. 209–233.

Clark, E., Hollon, E., LeBlanc, C., & Skinner, L. (2018) Assessment and Documentation in Child Life. In: Thompson, R. (ed.) *The Handbook of Child Life: A Guide for Pediatric Psychosocial Care*. Springfield, IL: Charles C Thomas.

Deavin, A., Greasley, P., & Dixon, C. (2018) Children's perspectives on living with a sibling with a chronic illness. *Pediatrics*, 142 (2), pp. e20174151.

Gaynard, L., & Jessee, P. (2018) The Paradigms of Play. In: Thompson, R. (ed.) *The Handbook of Child Life: A Guide for Pediatric Psychosocial Care*. Springfield, IL: Charles C Thomas.

Ginsburg, K. (2007) The importance of play in promoting healthy child development and maintaining strong parental-child bonds. *Pediatrics*, 119 (1), pp. 182–191.

Gordon, J., & Paisley, S. (2018) Trauma-Focused Medical Play. In: Rubin, L. (ed.) *Handbook of Medical Play Therapy and Child Life: Interventions in Clinical and Medical Settings*. Abingdon: Routledge.

Gursky, B. (2007) The effect of educational interventions with siblings of hospitalized children. *Journal of Developmental and Behavioral Pediatrics*, 28 (5), pp. 392–398.

Levick, J., Quinn, M., Holder, A., Nyberg, A., Beaumont, E., & Munch, S. (2010) Support for siblings of NICU patients: An interdisciplinary approach. *Social Work Health Care*, 49 (10), pp. 919–1033.

Masten, A. (2014) *Ordinary Magic: Resilience in Development*. New York, NY: Guilford Press.

Seymour, J. (2018) What About Me? Sibling Play Therapy when a Family Has a Child with Chronic Illness. In: Rubin, L. (ed.) *Handbook of Medical Play Therapy and Child Life: Interventions in Clinical and Medical Settings*. Abingdon: Routledge.

Turner, J. (2018) Theoretical Foundations of Child Life Practices. In: Thompson, R. (ed.) *The Handbook of Child Life: A Guide for Pediatric Psychosocial Care*. Springfield, IL: Charles C Thomas.

Woodburn, A., Munn, E., Jones, M., Hoskins, K., Gill, M., Fraser, C., Dunbar, J., Duplechain, A., Boles, J., & Bennett, K. (2020) *The Value of Certified Child Life Specialists: Direct and Downstream Optimization of Pediatric Patient and Family Outcomes*. Association of Child Life Professionals. [Online] Available from: <https://www.childlife.org/docs/default-source/the-child-life-profession/value-of-cclss-full-report.pdf> [Accessed 28 May 2022].

31

TAKING HOSPITAL PLAY INTO THE HOME

Tracy West – Oncology Outreach Play Specialist

"I couldn't do that job, I'd be crying all the time …" is one of the most frequent comments I hear from people when they ask me what I do as a profession. This chapter focuses on my role as an Outreach Play Specialist within children's oncology, particularly my more recent experiences of working with children, young people and their families receiving palliative care.

My first job as a play specialist was working within a medical/surgical ward where my main focus was on being able to help make a child's hospital experience as positive as possible. I used therapeutic play in a way that helped children understand their diagnosis and treatment and hopefully reduced any possible psychological trauma. This always resulted in them going home feeling better – that is, until I came to work in oncology … and then this changed.

I was the team leader on the oncology inpatient ward for ten years, working alongside other play leaders and play specialists. I loved the role but felt there were opportunities to explore and develop in the service we were providing. I took on a secondment for six months in order to scope and establish the Outreach Play Specialist role within the Macmillan team and was then successful in my application to take the role on full time. The role is funded by the amazing charity Candlelighters (2022), although I am employed by the National Health Service (NHS).

The scoping exercise found there were three main groups who were not able to access play support from within the hospital for various reasons. These were children experiencing extreme procedural anxiety, children receiving palliative care and siblings. These three groups have become the main focus of the role.

For the first couple of years I mainly worked with children who had severe procedural anxiety, mostly around portacath access and needles. However, over

DOI: 10.4324/9781003255444-37

the last few years the role has developed and changed direction, moving more towards working with children, young people and their families receiving palliative care, as well as supporting siblings through this difficult time. Siblings often become the forgotten child in a cancer diagnosis, not intentionally but due to circumstances out of the family's control. The work I do with siblings enables them to have some time that is just for them, and I aim to support them in understanding what is happening to their brother or sister, as well as giving them tools to cope in the future.

The hope is that all children diagnosed with cancer will be cured, sadly we know that is not the case. Each year children will die from cancer and many families are given the devastating news of a palliative diagnosis. In these circumstances surprisingly very little hospital intervention is required from this point and care is moved to the home or a hospice. When a family is told that their child's care is now palliative, life from that day will never be the same again.

Most people think palliative care means near the end of life. However, I often work with children and families for six to nine months and sometimes even longer before the child dies. Imagine having to live a life knowing this terrible outcome and not being able to change it, whilst also trying to make every day happy and memorable. This is where I am able to help and support the whole family within the home.

I have come to understand and learn with experience that all families are unique and one size does not fit all. Over the years I have worked with many children of different ages, genders, ethnic groups and with different beliefs. All these factors contribute to their palliative journey, end of life and the grieving process, which is what makes each and every family unique and individual. I therefore have to tailor my approach and methods to best suit those I am working with.

An example of how one size does not fit all is that in the same year I worked with two 11-year-old girls, both receiving palliative care, and who died within a month of each other. However, they each had very different journeys, and my support work with them was very different; the main difference being that one of the girls was aware of her diagnosis and prognosis right from the start and the other was not! The girl who knew her prognosis talked openly about dying and was involved in all conversations regarding her future. It was very clear that this was because of her faith and her strong belief as a Jehovah's Witness. During my sessions with her we were able to talk openly about death and this enabled her to choose all her own memory making keepsakes. She made things for her friends, Mum, brother and Dad. She was an amazing young girl, who didn't show any anger, fear or sadness about dying which I found remarkable and unbelievably brave of her. I worked with this family from diagnosis to death which was seven months of weekly visits. I remember doing handprints for jewellery and how openly we spoke about this being made for her Mum to keep her close.

The second girl had not engaged in conversations about her prognosis; she was not lied to or made to feel that she could not ask questions; she simply did not want to talk about it. Our sessions were tailored around doing nice activities together and we never spoke about death or her diagnosis during the sessions. We were able to make presents for occasions like Mother's Day and had lots of fun sessions that involved her best friend. Handprints for jewellery were done at the funeral directors, following her sad death.

I provided very different types of support on these occasions but that is not to say one was right or wrong. In both cases decisions were made by their parents who knew their child the best and made the best possible decisions they could at the time. It was a privilege to spend time with both girls and to be able to support them in doing these special things for both their families.

> Nothing we can do or say can take away the pain of bereavement, but families tell us of the importance of sensitive care. Poor care can intensify and prolong a family's distress, whilst care that is sensitive and appropriate can help families in their grief. The effects of this are positive and long-lasting.
>
> Supporting bereaved families includes good communication, responding to their needs in a timely way, and being emotionally self-aware.
>
> *Child Bereavement UK (2018)*

Memory making is a huge part of my role and with experience you come to learn that memory making is not just about hand and footprints or casts, but it is about spending time with a child and family and tailoring the mementos to specific family members so that it means something special (Figures 31.1–31.4). I remember doing tie dye with an 11-year-old boy who specifically chose to make a t-shirt for his older sister using her favourite colours. It was only after his death that his sister explained how important that t-shirt is to her and how wearing it brings her a sense of pride and closeness to him that she does not get from anything else. Memory making is different for all families, and I have to ensure that I provide equal opportunities for this whilst also respecting parent's decisions and choices.

I desperately wanted my daughter's hand and fingerprints but was emotionally unable to take them. Tracy again worked beyond our expectations and arranged with the funeral home to visit with me and did them on my behalf together. These were then made into a beautiful piece of artwork combining her and her sibling's handprints together. What a beautiful thing to have. The fingerprints were turned into jewellery and made very precious gifts. Candlelighters also funded a lady to make us some cushions and a unicorn, some wonderful keepsakes using her clothing, all items we can treasure.

As we reach the first anniversary of her passing, we have some really beautiful pieces to hold close, all of this and the memories that Tracy helped to create with her siblings. Tracy continues to play a huge part in our healing as a family and we can't thank her or Candlelighters enough.

Parent

We are all human and we would not be working in the caring professions if we did not care. Every palliative child and family that I work with has a lasting impact on me and I am truly sad when a precious life ends. I am often asked, "How do you find the strength and determination to be able to continue supporting other families?" Everyone has a different way of coping, and the way I look at it is that it is not my grief it is the family's, and although I am part of the journey it is not my journey.

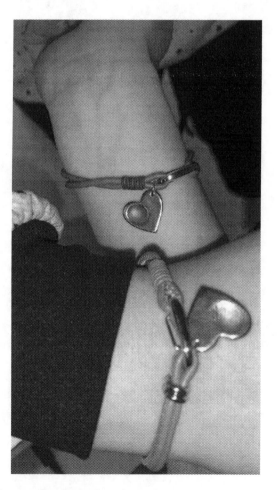

FIGURE 31.1 Memory fingerprint bracelets.

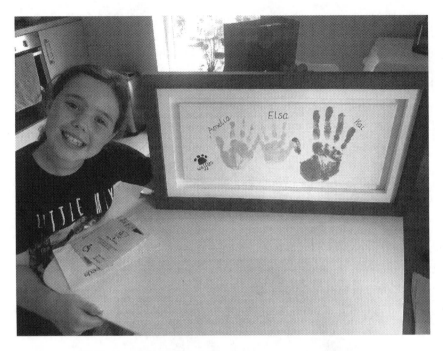

FIGURE 31.2 Sibling handprints framed.

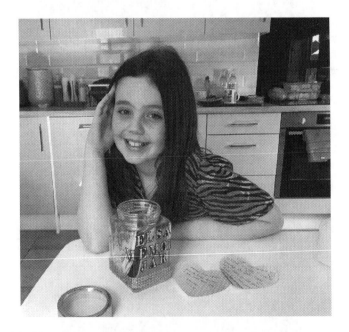

FIGURE 31.3 Memory jar.

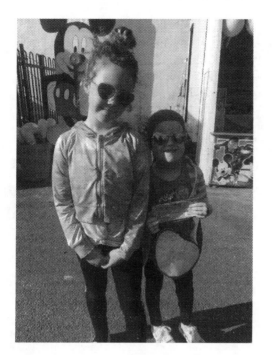

FIGURE 31.4 Siblings.

When I first started this role, if someone had told me about some of the conversations I would be having with parents about death and some of the situations I would be in, I would certainly have thought twice about taking on the role. However, five years on and these conversations feel like the most natural thing to me because they are part of how I support each family. I remember visiting a family after their son's death and having a cup of tea in his bedroom, us chatting away and her beautiful boy lying in bed on the cold mattress. His mum had said it did not feel right us being downstairs and him being upstairs because that would never have happened when I visited as my time was always spent with her child. I consider this to be a huge privilege.

Conversations about a child's death are extremely sensitive and difficult to have with parents. At first I could not imagine how they would go and did not know how to even get started, but with experience I learnt that these conversations happen at the family's own pace and when they feel they can trust you. When they do, they feel very natural and comfortable because the parent has opened up to you (Figures 31.5–31.8). For some parents this is quite soon after diagnosis and usually due to them worrying about how to talk to siblings. However, sometimes this is very near the end of life and even sometimes isn't until after death. There is no right or wrong way but is again all individual to each family's journey. Being respectful of their decisions is paramount to me being able to develop a supportive relationship and the success of my role within the family.

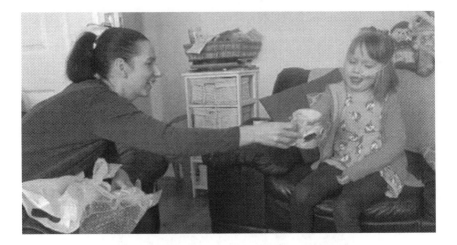

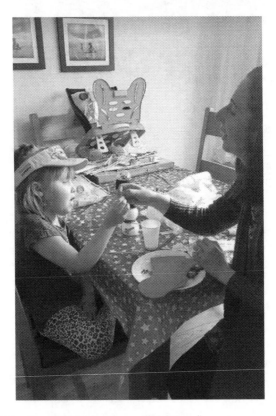

FIGURES 31.5–31.8 Fun activities at home. *(Continued)*

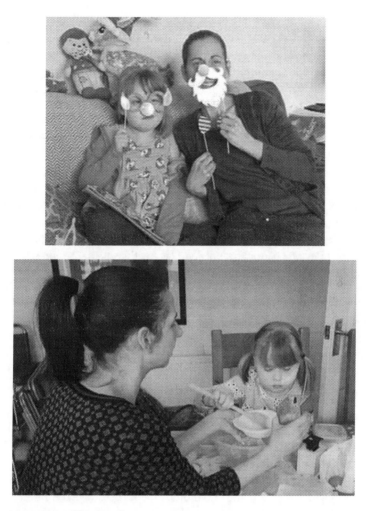

FIGURES 31.5–31.8 *(Continued)*

When my healthy happy middle child was diagnosed, out of the blue, with a terminal brain cancer (DIPG) – our world and hearts were shattered. How can you be told there is nothing to save your six-year-old daughter – basically just go home and make memories. It all feels so wrong and hopeless and so very lonely and dark. You soon realise that the only thing that matters then is to make sure your dying child is protected and feels nothing but love, joy and happiness, in whatever time they have left. We met many different medical staff and teams who were there to help our daughter and ourselves. From neurology and oncology nurses and consultants to the amazing radiotherapy team, the hardworking Macmillan team, to the fantastic play specialists and many more. Every single one played a very important part of our "journey" with her cancer and demise. All so very vital to her care and well-being but the one who brought the most smiles, laughter, happiness and positive distractions for her was Tracy West, her outreach play specialist. She was there from the very beginning, making scary appointments and check-ups and procedures lighter and less scary. When we were broken and drained from caring for her 24/7, Tracy would visit us at home and spend hours playing with her, making her happy whilst we had some quick respite. Whilst she was stuck at home and her brother and sister were at school learning and thriving, Tracy made her feel special when she felt left out and not normal.

Tracy supported myself with what to say when my other children asked questions about their beloved sister dying and what would happen. Growing and building an important relationship with my other two children, in the run up to her death and the aftermath so they had someone external who they could speak to who was part of their sister's last months. She helped bring my grieving children support and care within the home and school to bring them a relaxed, fun and safe place to speak about their sister and their feelings dealing with their grief and massive loss. Helping them remember what they loved about her and making thoughtful crafts and souvenirs with them to focus on the happiness and love they shared together.

To me this is the most precious source of support, especially when there's no fix, no cure and no hope. Tracy always brought joy during the darkest of times. We will never forget what she did for our angel and our family.

Parent

No one can change the outcome for these children and their families, but I pride myself on being able to support them in even the smallest of ways that will make a positive difference, if not now, but in the future. I consider myself extremely privileged and honoured to work within this role. Yes, it is difficult and extremely sad at times, but I hold on to the fact that I make a difference to the families at the most unimaginably difficult time. I feel like my professional career has been leading up to this role and I could not imagine doing anything else now. It is a privilege to be invited into a family's home, and to be able to share some of their remaining time with their child is a real honour.

Huge thank you to Candlelighters (2022) for supporting this much needed and essential role.

References

Candlelighters (2022) *Home Page* – [Online] Available from: <https://www.candlelighters.org.uk/> [Accessed 11 December 2022]

Child Bereavement UK (2018) Supporting Bereaved Families. [Online] Available from: <https://www.childbereavementuk.org/pages/category/working-with-bereaved-families> [Accessed 4 April 2022]

32

CONCLUDING THOUGHTS

*Nicky Everett – Senior Lecturer and Health
Play Specialist*

Cath Hubbuck – Senior Health Play Specialist

The aim of this book was to explore the real-life perspectives of those play practitioners working within healthcare with children and young people, examining how play can aid and support them during this potentially difficult time. In an ideal world children would not spend any time within hospital, dealing with sickness or trauma but for many children this **is** their real-life experience. In this situation a child's need for play is still essential, but it also increases and changes, and how those play needs are met, changes too. In hospital children experience many things that are far beyond their current development and understanding of the world. They are potentially separated from family, friends, school, community, and everything familiar and they must cope very quickly with many new, unfamiliar, and unsettling experiences. They may encounter many new adults and have to undergo strange and distressing examinations or procedures.

In these circumstances play becomes a powerful and effective tool for helping children to navigate their way through this new environment. Play can allow for restoration of control at a time when all aspects of life may be out of control. It provides ways of communicating and understanding an adult-centric clinical world of healthcare and brings some comfort and familiarity in the face of what could be potentially, very stressful circumstances. To be a Health Play Specialist is to care and to help children and their families through challenging times and to do it all with an approach that upholds play, exudes joy, and encourages exploration and curiosity throughout it all.

By examining the diverse work of play practitioners within healthcare, it is clear how complex this role can be, but also how rewarding it can be. It is an honour to accompany a family's journey, providing some incredibly rewarding moments during a time which can only be described as an emotional roller-coaster for all involved. The play team inhabit a unique role where they

DOI: 10.4324/9781003255444-38

provide nonclinical relief, from the experience children have in hospital, whilst also being part of the clinical multidisciplinary team. Play is often the bridge between the two.

Our contributors have demonstrated the importance of conversations with parents, young people, and children, for example about death and dying. This is often undertaken by Play Specialists and is a skill acquired by experience and cannot be learnt from a textbook, course, or study day. Play is such an important element of a child's life, and this should not be paused or stopped due to a hospital admission, but rather it bridges communication with healthcare professionals and supports successful adaptation within an environment where they have little control. In acknowledging and utilising the power of play, play teams can help children to learn about different procedures and treatments, whilst creating a positive and supportive environment.

We are incredibly grateful for our international contributors who have given us a valuable insight into hospital play services and the training of practitioner around the world. These international perspectives have highlighted the challenges faced in the integration of play into the clinical environment of the hospitals. They have shown diversity in their approach and practice but ultimately, we share the same goals, which are to help sick children through play and to advocate for their needs when they are unable to do so themselves.

Collectively, the chapters of this book – drawn together from play specialist, child life specialist, and therapeutic play experts from all around the world – have demonstrated many of the ways in which play staff in hospitals undertake this extraordinary work, in extraordinary environments and often under extraordinary pressure. It is often perceived that the role of play in hospital is unimportant or a passive activity to prevent boredom or to keep children quiet and happy. In actual fact it is so much more than this and not necessarily what people might think at all. There is a serious side and – in the moment – there is often an urgency to the work of play staff, especially when they are involved in clinical procedures. This role requires personal and professional resilience; it is challenging working with very distressed and sick children, it is equally necessary to stay calm in the moment while processing each encounter as it happens, in an ever-changing environment.

What is evident within the chapters of this book is that the role of the play team is so much more than just a Job Description or a professional title and the variance in practice is very wide. Play staff work hard to become experts in their field of practice and to know the best ways to meet the needs of children receiving health care. As practitioners who know and understand children and child development, as well as the impact of illness and hospitalisation, they strive to uphold play and keep this at the centre of all their interactions with children, young people – and sometimes even adult patients too. There does seem to be a significant lack of understanding about the importance of play for children in healthcare settings and the work of health play staff themselves. There is a great need for further rigorous research into the impact of play and the experience of sick children in healthcare settings, along with how the skills of the play team can be better utilised by the wider multidisciplinary team.

This work is about addressing children's distress and trauma, and connecting them with normality through the medium of play. For a child there is nothing as normal as playing. We must not forget that, just because they happen to be in a healthcare environment.

APPENDIX

Useful internet references

Academy of Play and Child Psychotherapy (APAC) – https://apac.org.uk/
American Journal of Play – https://www.museumofplay.org/journalofplay/
Association for the Study of Play – https://studyofplay.org/
Charter for Children's Play – https://www.playengland.org.uk/charter-for-play
Fair Play for Children – https://fairplayforchildren.org/
Healthcare Play Specialist Education Trust – https://hpset.org.uk/
International Journal of Play – https://www.tandfonline.com/journals/rijp20
International Play Association – https://ipaworld.org/
Leeds Beckett University Childhood Development and Playwork BA (Hons) degree course –
    https://www.leedsbeckett.ac.uk/courses/childhood-development-playwork-ba
Milly's Smiles – https://www.millyssmiles.org/
National Association of Health Play Specialists – https://www.nahps.org.uk/
Play Board Northern Ireland – https://www.playboard.org/
Play England – https://www.playengland.org.uk/
Play Scotland – https://www.playscotland.org/
Play Therapy UK – https://playtherapy.org.uk/
Play Wales – https://www.playwales.org.uk/eng/
Starlight Children's Foundation – https://www.starlight.org/

INDEX

Note: *Italicised* folios refers figures.

Printed in the United States
by Baker & Taylor Publisher Services